PICKLE PLEDGE

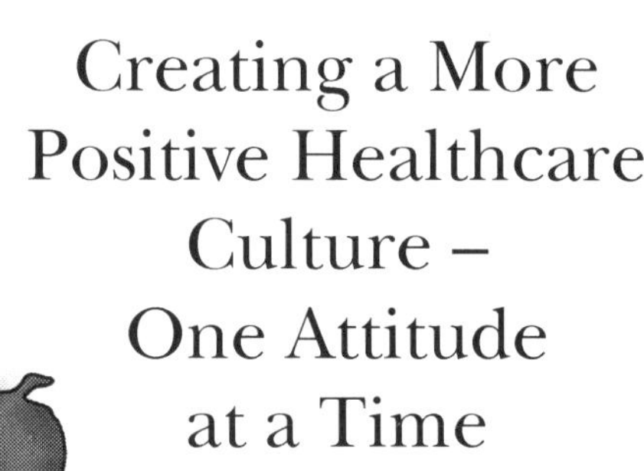

Creating a More Positive Healthcare Culture – One Attitude at a Time

Featuring The Pickle Challenge for Charity

JOE TYE & BOB DENT

Joe Tye is CEO and Head Coach at Values Coach Inc. He can be reached at Joe@ValuesCoach.com

Bob Dent is Senior Vice President of Midland Health and COO/CNO of Midland Memorial Hospital in Midland, Texas. He can be reached at Bob.Dent@Midland-Memorial.com. See also, www.DrBobDent.com.

For additional resources and to see examples of The Pickle Pledge and The Pickle Challenge for Charity in action go to www.TheFlorenceChallenge.com/Pickle

ISBN#: 1-88751139-3
ISBN 13#: 978-1-887511-39-1

Book design by Studio 6 Sense • studio6sense.com

Front cover illustration by Vern Herschberger

Big Pickle chainsaw carving by Don Hill; photograph by Laura Isbell

For Michelle and Kim, who make us leave our pickles
in the parking lot when we come to work,
and for Sally and Karen, who make us leave our pickles
in the driveway when we come home.

Advance Praise for Pickle Pledge

"I promise this book will delight and refresh you! We've employed the thought provoking, practical approaches in our organization and truly reenergized our culture of care!"

Nancy Howell Agee, RN, MSN
President and CEO Carilion Clinic

"Every day leaders have the opportunity to inspire staff to embrace human caring passionately as they perform their duties. The Pickle Pledge is an excellent, easy to comprehend and must read for all seeking to create and sustain healthy environments that support human caring for our patients and colleagues."

Linda Burnes Bolton, DrPH, RN, FAAN
Cedars-Sinai Chief Nursing Executive
Past President, American Organization of Nurse Executives

"This book is profound and helps to create a personal and professional life changing experience for leaders and for the entire workforce. The authors give a framework for change and sustainability in order to create a workplace environment that is positive, truthful and caring. I was completely engrossed in the learnings from this book and stimulated to make changes within myself in order to improve the professional and personal world in which I practice!!!!"

Rhonda Anderson, DNSc, RN, FAAN, FACHE
President, RMA Consulting
Past President, American Organization of Nurse Executives

"Change begins with you, as real happiness springs from within and this practical and actionable guide to de-pickling and pickling prevention is an inspired way to begin any transformation. Healthcare needs more cultures of respect, that value difference and strive for inclusion where we show up as our best selves. Our patients deserve that, our peers deserve that, and you deserve that. Take The Pickle Pledge!"

Dr. Cole Edmonson DNP, RN, FACHE, NEA-BC
Chief Nursing Officer, Administration
Texas Health

"Every moment of the day I aspire to stage the best possible experience for those around me. The Pickle Pledge is a great tool to stage the best possible experience for everyone. This book offers a fun, easy and effective way to create a culture of greatness."

Sylvain Trepanier, DNP, RN, CENP
System Chief Nursing Officer

"We have the opportunity as leaders to not only create a culture where staff enjoy coming to work, but are passionate about maintaining a drama-free, emotionally healthy environment – the sort of Pickle-Free Zone described by the authors. This book contains invaluable lessons that I have used to create and maintain a culture of ownership in our facility which has helped us attract and retain great people."

Michelle Turner RN, BSN, Nurse Manager
University of Iowa Hospitals and Clinics, Iowa River Landing

About the Authors

Joe Tye is Founder, CEO and Head Coach of Values Coach Inc., which provides consulting, coaching and training on organizational culture and values-based life and leadership skills for healthcare clients. Joe earned a Master's Degree in Hospital and Health Administration from The University of Iowa and an MBA from the Stanford Graduate School of Business, where he was class co-president. He is the author of 12 books, including *The Florence Prescription: From Accountability to Ownership,* which has nearly 500,000 copies in print. Prior to founding Values Coach in 1994 Joe was chief operating officer for several large community teaching hospitals. On the volunteer front he was founding president of the Association of Air Medical Services and as founder of STAT (Stop Teenage Addiction to Tobacco) was a leading activist fighting against unethical tobacco industry marketing practices. He and his wife Sally have two adult children. They live on a small farmstead in Iowa and their second home is a tent in the Grand Canyon.

Bob Dent is Senior Vice President of Midland Health and Chief Operating Officer / Chief Nursing Officer at Midland Memorial Hospital. Bob has more than 27 years as a nurse and healthcare leader. His honors and awards include: *Modern Healthcare's* Class of 2006 Up and Comers in Healthcare Administration; the Texas Organization of Nurse Executives 2013 Excellence in Leadership Awardee; and the 2014 Texas Tech University Health Sciences Center's Distinguished Alumni where he earned his doctorate degree in nursing practice. He is passionate about the professional practice of nursing and leadership. Outside of work, Bob enjoys being with his wife, five children and two grandchildren. You might find him in the garden or on the racquetball court, where he is a fierce competitor!

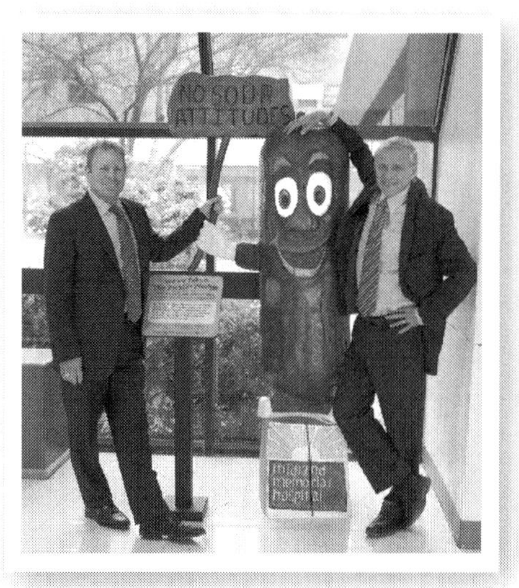

Joe and Bob with the Positive Mr. Pickle at the employee entrance of Midland Memorial Hospital

Other books by Joe Tye

The Florence Prescription: From Accountability to Ownership

All Hands on Deck: 8 Essential Lessons for Building a Culture of Ownership

The Cultural Blueprinting Toolkit Workbook

Leadership Lessons from The Hobbit and The Lord of the Rings

The Twelve Core Action Values

The Healing Tree: A Mermaid, A Poet, and A Miracle

Pioneer Spirit, Caring Heart, Healing Mission

The Farmer

Winning the War with Yourself Field Manual

Staying on Top When Your World's Upside Down

Your Dreams Are Too Small

Never Fear, Never Quit: A Story of Courage and Perseverance

Everyday Courage for Extraordinary Times

Coming Spring 2017

Watch for Joe's and Bob's next book – *Building a Culture of Ownership in Healthcare: The Invisible Architecture of Core Values, Attitude, and Self-Empowerment* – coming from Sigma Theta Tau International in Spring of 2017

The Pickle Pledge
"I will turn
every complaint
into either a
blessing or a
constructive
suggestion"
Be a
POSITIVE
PICKLE

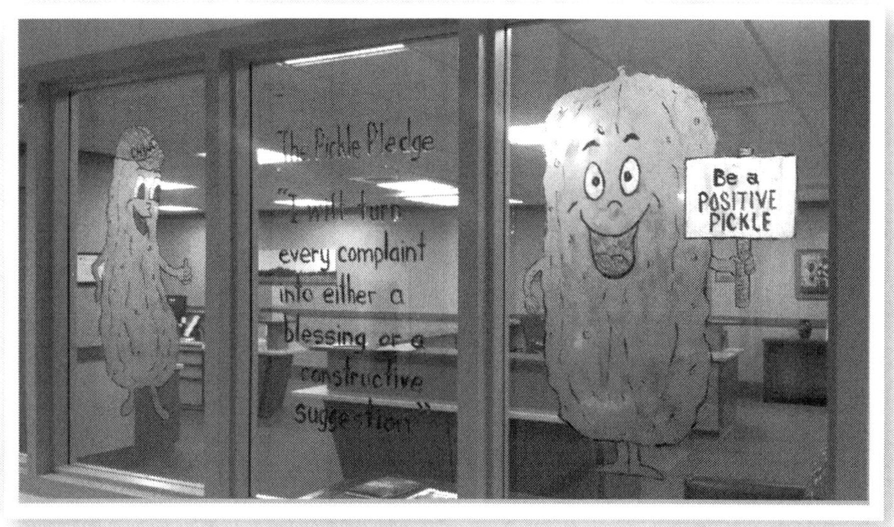

Administrative offices at Community Hospitals and Wellness Centers, Bryan, Ohio

PICKLE PLEDGE

Creating a More Positive Healthcare Culture – One Attitude at a Time

By Joe Tye and Bob Dent

"Prying into one another's concerns, acting behind another's back, backbiting, misrepresentation, bad temper, bad thoughts, murmuring, complaining. Do we ever think of how we bear the responsibility for all the harm that we cause in this way?"

Florence Nightingale in a letter to graduates
of the Nightingale School of Nursing

"One toxically negative person can drag down morale and productivity of an entire work unit. It is a leadership responsibility to create a workplace environment where toxic emotional negativity is not tolerated."

Joe Tye: *The Florence Prescription:*
From Accountability to Ownership

"I got a whole new team and didn't have to change the people because they changed themselves."

Paul Utemark, Chief Executive Officer
Fillmore County Health System
Geneva, Nebraska

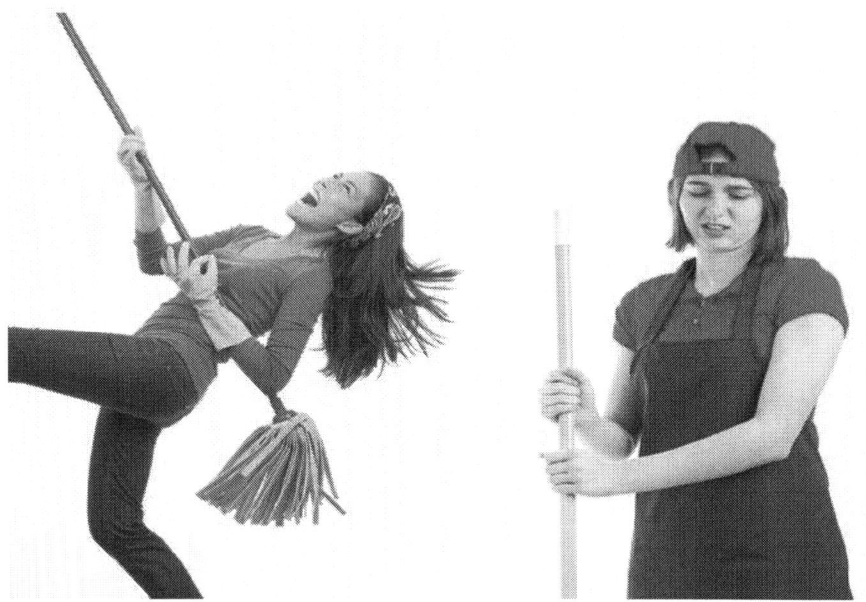

Same job, different attitude.

Who do you think is happier?

Who would you rather work with?

Who would you rather live with?

Who is going to be a better parent?

Who is going to be a better friend?

Who is more likely to be promoted at work?

Who would you rather be like?

Definitions

Pickle-Sucker: A person who frequently complains, often about trivial matters, so-called because at least metaphorically speaking chronic complainers have the facial expression of someone who has just tasted a sour dill pickle. While even the most positive of people can on occasion have a pickle-sucker day, when it persists the term becomes synonymous with emotional vampire.

Pickle-Free Zone: Any area of the organization, or of the home, that is off-limits to petty whining and complaining, gossip and rumor-mongering, and intimidating or bullying behavior.

The Pickle Pledge: A simple (though not always easy) promise that one makes to turn complaints into *blessings* by replacing resentment with gratitude, and into *constructive suggestions* by replacing passivity with initiative.

The Pickle Challenge for Charity: A one-week period when people make a commitment to turn complaints into contributions by placing a quarter (or an IOU) into a decorated pickle jar every time they catch themselves, or are caught by a coworker, engaging in toxic emotional negativity (see next definition), with proceeds being donated to a worthwhile charity. The Pickle Challenge for Charity is often the spark for impressive culture change within the organization as well as dramatic personal change for individuals who take it seriously.

Toxic Emotional Negativity (TEN): While not yet officially listed in the International Statistical Classification of Diseases and Related Health Problems, toxic emotional negativity (TEN) is increasingly recognized as being seriously detrimental to human health and happiness for both the toxically negative person him or herself and for those upon whom TEN is inflicted in the form of chronic complaining, gossiping and rumor-mongering, bullying and lateral violence.

The other BMW Club: A group of people who collectively engage in toxic emotional negativity by bitching, moaning, whining and complaining together. Often accompanied by commiseration (see next definition).

Commiseration: To co-miserate, or be miserable together.

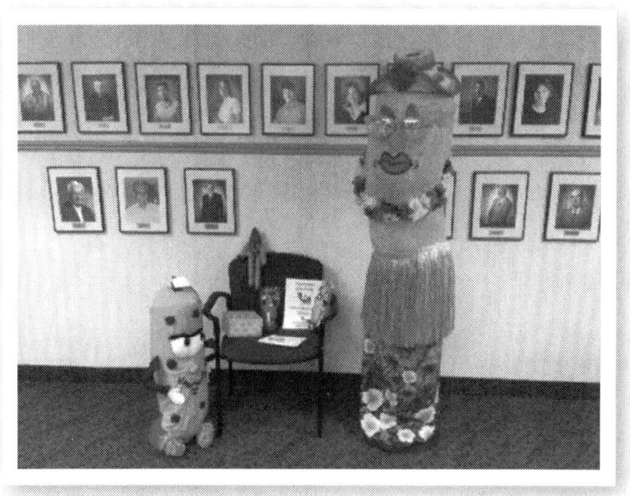

The Big Pickle at Sidney Regional Medical Center, Sidney, Nebraska

Contents

Part 1
Emotionally Healthy Healthcare

The Promise that Will Change Your Life

I've Taken The Pickle Pledge

"I will turn every complaint into either a blessing or constructive suggestion."

By taking **The Pickle Pledge**, I am promising myself that I will no longer waste my time and energy on blaming, complaining, and gossiping, nor will I commiserate with those who steal my energy with their blaming, complaining, and gossiping.

* So-called because chronic complainers look like they were born with a dill pickle stuck in their mouths.

ValuesCoach.com • TheFlorenceChallenge.com

The twin commitments to *gratitude* and *initiative* that are embedded within The Pickle Pledge will change your perspective on every problem, obstacle, or challenge you face in your life. You will stop letting petty grievances, real or imagined, drain the energy, joy, and spunk from your life. You will start thinking more creatively about how to solve problems and not just complain about them. When you take The Pickle Pledge you are effectively dropping your membership in what we call "the *other* BMW Club" – Bitching, Moaning, Whining and Complaining.

It's called The Pickle Pledge because people who are always whining and complaining look like they've been sucking on a dill pickle, at least metaphorically speaking. It's also appropriate because a pickle is a fresh cucumber that's been soaked in vinegar, and isn't that sort of what it feels like to be around someone who is always complaining – like they've been soaked in vinegar?

There is, of course, one big difference between a human pickle and the kind you find on the grocery store shelves. A grocery store pickle can never be turned back into a fresh cucumber. But humans *can* transform. All they need to do is make different choices about their attitudes towards life and towards other people.

You can download The Pickle Pledge mini-poster at www.TheFlorenceChallenge.com/Pickle

Creating an Emotionally Healthy Workplace

This is a Pickle Free Zone
PLEASE!
Leave your Gossiping, Complaining, Criticizing, and Toxic Emotional Negativity at the door.
THANK YOU!
ValuesCoach.com • TheFlorenceChallenge.com

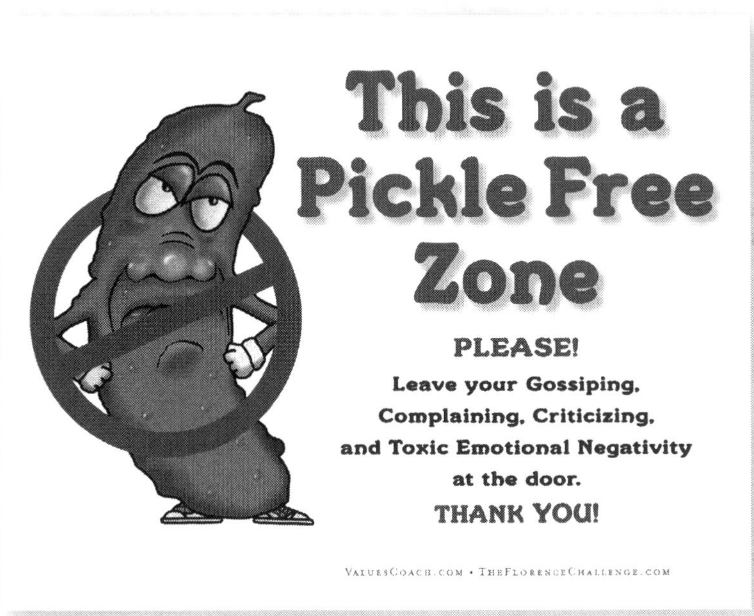

People should have the right to a workplace that is free from fear, free from bullying, free from gossip and rumor-mongering, and free from chronic complaining and other forms of TEN. And managers have a responsibility to support their people by declaring the workplace to be a Pickle-Free Zone (PFZ) the way we once had to protect the health of workers by declaring the workplace to be a smoke-free zone. A PFZ is any area of the workplace – or of the home – where TEN is not wanted or welcome. This does not mean that people aren't permitted to identify, talk about, and deal with real and legitimate problems – quite to the contrary. It only means that they are not welcome to whine about them.

You can download a Pickle-Free Zone mini-poster at www.TheFlorenceChallenge.com/Pickle

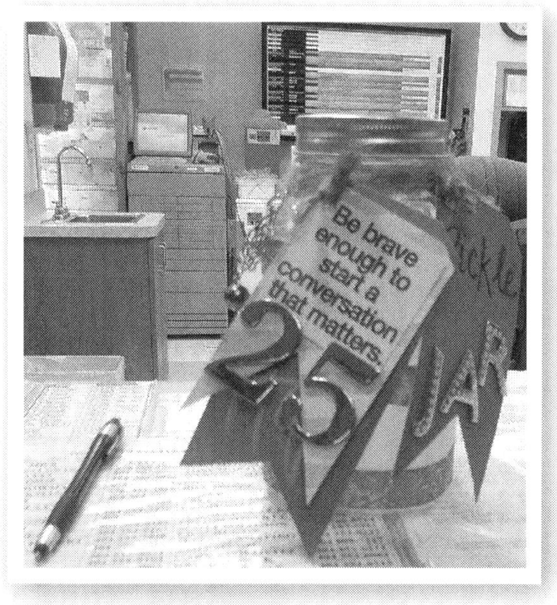

The Challenge that Will Transform Your Organization

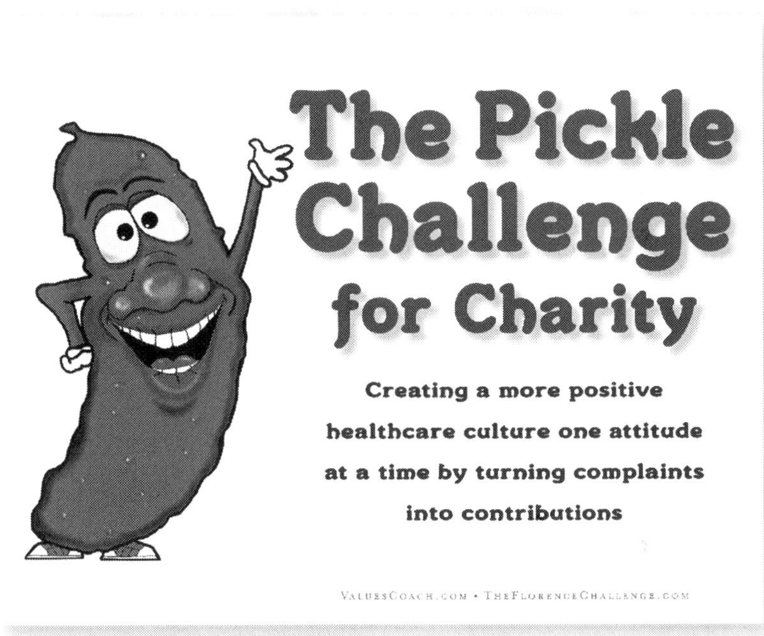

The Pickle Challenge for Charity
Creating a more positive healthcare culture one attitude at a time by turning complaints into contributions
ValuesCoach.com • TheFlorenceChallenge.com

The Pickle Challenge for Charity is a one-week period when everyone in your organization is encouraged to drop a quarter (or an IOU) into a decorated pickle jar whenever they catch themselves, or are caught by coworkers, engaging in emotional negativity. Prior to the weeklong event a variety of activities – including a Culture Assessment Survey, pickle jar decorating and cake making contests, poster displays, and other activities create anticipation and enthusiasm for the event. At the event's conclusion, all pickle jar proceeds, along with any matching funds that have been committed, are donated to the charity selected by the organization.

You can see examples of the incredibly creative things being done for The Pickle Challenge for Charity at www.TheFlorenceChallenge.com/Pickle

Transforming an Organization: The Midland Memorial Hospital Story

When Midland Memorial Hospital (MMH) opened a magnificent new $176 million patient care tower in late 2012, there was every expectation that patient satisfaction would soar. Indeed, a big part of the motivation for building the new tower had been to deal with patient satisfaction scores that were so low the hospital's leadership team had actually been cited by its accrediting body for not taking appropriate action to improve their scores. The new facility was beautiful and designed with patients, families, and staff members in mind. Among other things, MMH was one of the first hospitals in the nation to have ceiling-mounted automatic lifts with motors installed over every bed so that no nurse would ever suffer a back injury from trying to lift a patient. The full-service cafeteria offers a wide range of gourmet and healthy food choice options. There is a beautiful courtyard accessible to patients, staff and visitors with a full-size walking labyrinth and patient care floors are designed to assure optimal nursing care.

Unfortunately, not only did patient satisfaction fail to increase, it actually continued to slide. By the end of 2013 it had reached record low levels. Just as concerning, there was evidence that employee engagement had not been improved by the new building. It quickly became clear what the problem had been: by opening this gorgeous new facility, MMH had raised expectations, but by moving in the same old culture, attitudes, and behaviors had increased rather than decreased the gap between new and higher expectations and the actual experience of working or receiving care in that new facility.

At the beginning of 2014 MMH, working with Values Coach, launched a far-reaching Values and Culture Initiative focused on the organization's Invisible Architecture of core values, organizational culture, and workplace attitude. Using a construction metaphor, the hospital's leadership team created a cultural blueprint in which the foundation is core values, the superstructure is organizational culture, and the interior finish is workplace attitude. In the process, the culture has evolved from one where the focus was on accountability to one where the focus is on ownership.

The results have been remarkable. MMH came into 2014 with record low employee engagement and patient satisfaction and by the end of the year both measures were at a record high, and have been steadily increasing ever since. Improved employee engagement has had a positive impact on clinical quality outcomes and on determinants of value-based purchasing. The hospital's image and reputation in the community and in surrounding regions has significantly improved, a fact reflected in the tone of letters received from patients and family members. Following are results from follow-up Culture Assessment Surveys:

» 63% of responding employees agreed or strongly agreed that their coworkers were more positive and fully engaged than before the start of the Values and Culture Initiative.

» 87% of responding employees agreed or strongly agreed that they were personally more aware of their own attitudes and the attitudes of people around them, and were more fully engaged in their work, than before the start of the Values and Culture Initiative.

- 94% of managers agreed or strongly agreed that the Values and Culture Initiative has helped them to be both personally and professionally more effective.
- 92% of graduates from the first series of courses on The Twelve Core Action Values said that they would recommend the course to others, and more than one-third called the course life-changing.
- The percentage of employees agreeing or strongly agreeing that their coworkers refrain from complaining and other forms of toxic emotional negativity, and treat others with respect, increased from 36% to 61%.
- A substantial percentage of employee paid hours were shifted from complaining, gossiping and other forms of toxic emotional negativity into working with patients, communicating between departments, and investing in personal and professional skills development, resulting in an annual Cultural Productivity Benefit of $7.2 million.
- In May of 2016, as a result of the impressive culture transformation that had occurred over the previous three years, Midland Health was the first organization to earn the INSPIRED Award for Values and Culture Excellence from Values Coach.

The essential first step in the MMH cultural transformation journey was to assess and acknowledge the magnitude of toxic emotional negativity (TEN) within the organization and then to launch The Pickle Challenge for Charity to raise awareness and change behavior.

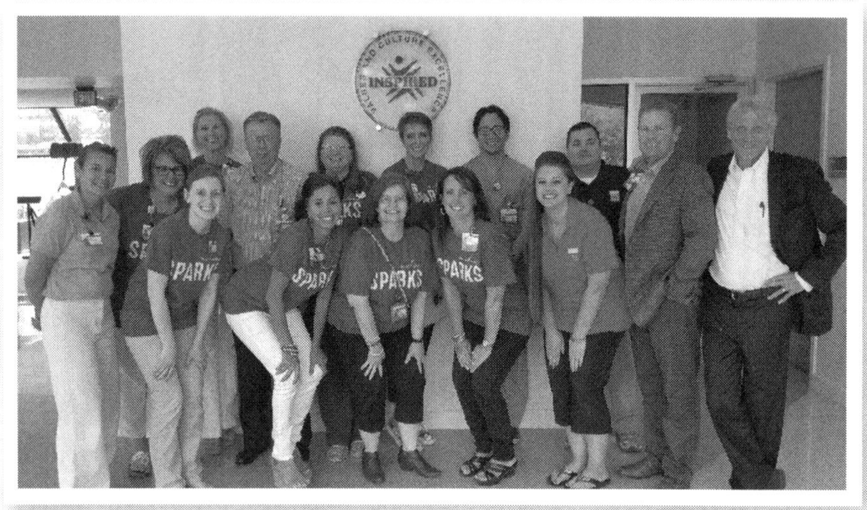

Some of MMH's Certified Values Coach Trainers with the INSPIRED Award for Values and Culture Excellence

---

Several weeks after Midland Memorial Hospital completed the Pickle Challenge for Charity, DNV accreditation surveyors showed up. During their summation, all three surveyors – the nurse, the physician, and the administrator – commented on how much more positive the culture was than it had been on their last visit. All three mentioned the decorated pickle jars they'd seen all around the facility. And the nurse surveyor said that the highlight of her week had been when she'd heard a nurse tell a physician that he was being a pickle and invited him to deposit a quarter in the unit's pickle jar. And he did!

Personal Transformation – Why we wrote this book

We both absolutely believe in the power of The Pickle Pledge to help people change their lives for the better, and in the power of The Pickle Challenge for Charity to help organizations foster a more positive and productive culture of ownership. We've seen it work – and work beautifully – at Midland Health and at many other organizations. But we both have more deeply personal reasons for writing this book. Here are our stories.

Bob's Story

In September of 2015, I was admitted to Midland Memorial Hospital, where I serve as Chief Operating Officer and Chief Nursing Officer, with acute chest pain. Two years before I'd had a stent and then a two vessel cardiac bypass surgery. I was told that one of my bypass grafts had closed and that I now required a stent placement at a location that made it a very high-risk surgery. I was told that if the vessel dissected during the surgery I would have to be transferred by helicopter to Dallas – that is, if I lived through it.

I had everything to live for: a family I love dearly and children who are my pride and joy; a great job where I'm privileged to work with amazing colleagues; high-level involvement in multiple professional associations and local service organizations; and being part of a community where "West Texas Friendly" is more than just a slogan. The prospect of losing all that, and losing it so suddenly, was frightening and depressing.

By that time, I'd been repeating The Pickle Pledge and each day's promise from The Self Empowerment Pledge for so long that I didn't just know the words by heart – they popped up in my mind instantaneously. It was almost as if a great wall had been erected to hold back anxiety, worry and depression. I took a deep breath and reminded myself of how grateful I was to be in a place where I could receive the care I needed, and that following the surgery there would be actions I could take to prevent any recurrence. The rest I left in God's hands.

Joe and I started working on this book almost a year after that surgery. In the intervening months I have met with members of the Midland Memorial Hospital staff every morning at 8:16 sharp for our Daily Leadership Huddle. Every day we start with the group reciting The Pickle Pledge and that day's promise from The Self Empowerment Pledge. Like me, most of the participants no longer need to read the promises, they know them by heart. Our story was reported in *H&HN Daily*, a publication of the American Hospital Association.

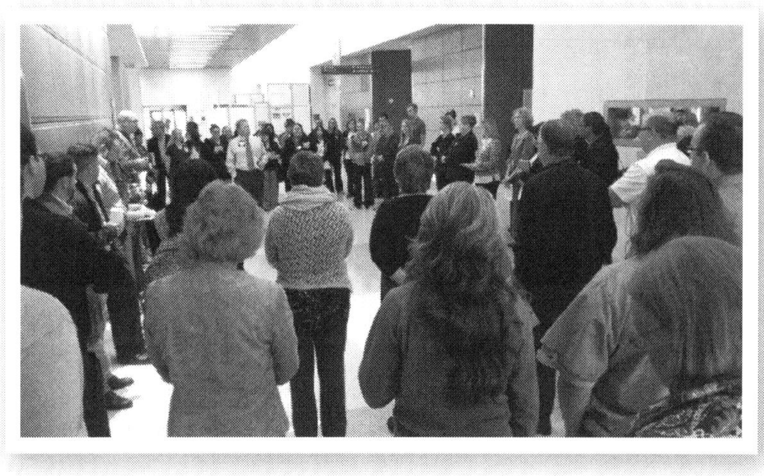

The Daily Leadership Huddle at Midland Memorial Hospital

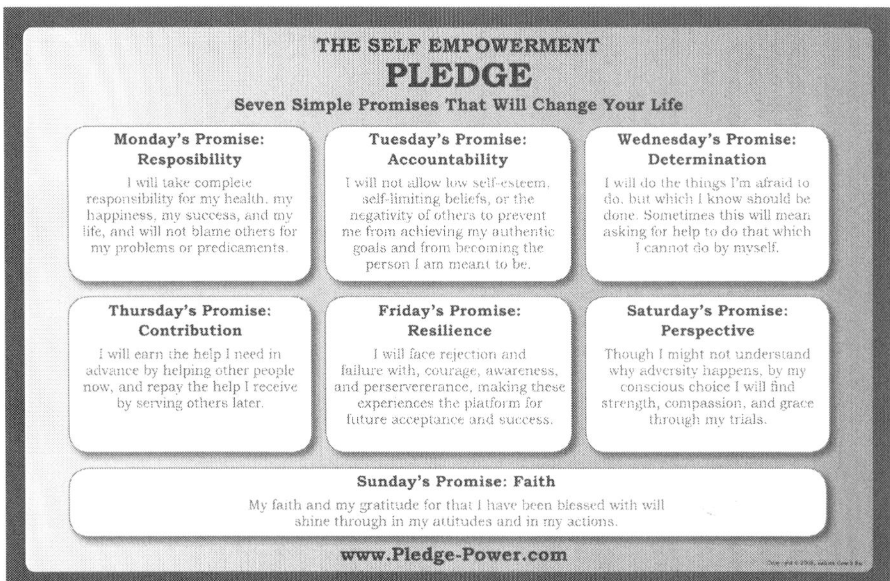

The 7 Promises of The Self Empowerment Pledge

Learn more about the 21-module advanced PledgePower course on The Self Empowerment Pledge at www.PledgePower.com.

JOE'S STORY

One Sunday in late October of 2015, I boarded a plane bound for Texas. I was scheduled to meet with the executive leadership team of Otto Kaiser Memorial Hospital in Kenedy that evening, and then over the next three days help them work on what we call the Invisible Architecture of core values, organizational culture, and workplace attitude; at the time they were in the final stages of completing the visible architecture for a new replacement hospital facility, and wanted to make sure that what into that beautiful new building was just as beautiful. At least that was the plan. I arrived with classic symptoms of acute appendicitis and after a short meeting with the executive team in the board room was escorted to the emergency room. A CT scan ruled out appendicitis and ruled in acute diverticulitis; I was admitted as an inpatient, and for the next three days received exemplary care.

The following Thursday morning I was discharged in time to catch my scheduled flight back home with instructions to check in with my family physician as soon as I landed. I was to continue with a regimen of oral antibiotics and the next Monday fly to Pennsylvania for a special nursing retreat at WellSpan Health System. From there I was headed for Huron, South Dakota for three days at Huron Regional Medical Center. At least that was the plan.

That evening found me in the Emergency Treatment Center of the University of Iowa Hospitals and Clinics (some 35 years previously I'd begun my hospital administration career as manager of that very department). I was once again admitted. Four days into my inpatient stay the senior surgery resident came into my room and told me that what they were doing wasn't working and that the next step would be to have part of my colon removed. That would also mean that I'd have to wear a colostomy bag for up to a year following the surgery, and possibly for the rest of my life. I told her that I would rather die. She smiled and said that we should explore other options than dying.

Every now and then, life presents you with a moment of truth. There is a fork in the road – an unexpected adversity or opportunity – and you have a choice to make, perhaps one of the most significant choices you will ever make. The most important part of that choice is often not the decision itself, it's the attitude with which you make that decision. I looked at the wall where I had taped up The Pickle Pledge. Then I looked up at the IV pole where I'd draped my wristbands for each of the 7 promises of The Self Empowerment Pledge.

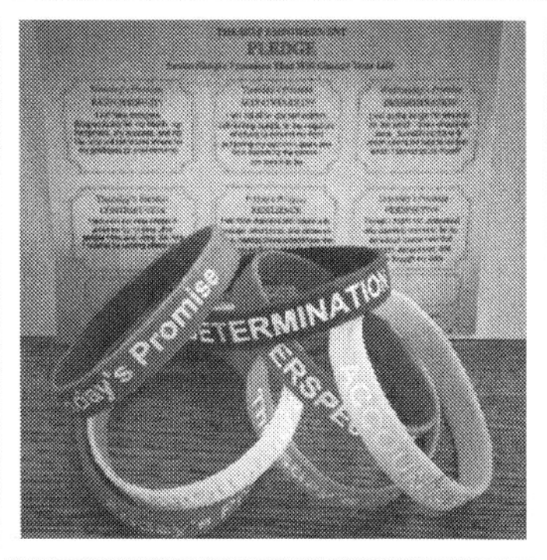

Over the next three hours I fought an intense inner battle. It would have been easy for me to feel sorry for myself and allow myself to slip into "poor me" victim mode. Later that evening I said a prayer of thanksgiving for the incredible care I had received at two very different hospitals more than a thousand miles apart. Then I grabbed my IV pole and started walking. For the next five days I walked up and down the corridors of that hospital (one of the nurses told me that I should enter the IV pole Olympics). As I walked, I talked to my colon, promising that I was going to take much better care of it in the future. Five days later I walked out of the hospital with my colon intact. The following January I made up all three programs that had been cancelled because of my health scare. And I am trying very hard to keep the promises that I made to my colon.

“People don’t quit a mission, they will only quit a job.
People don’t leave a team, they will only leave an organization.
People don’t desert a leader, they will only desert a boss.”

Joe Tye: *All Hands on Deck: 8 Essential Lessons for Building a Culture of Ownership*

WHY WE WANT YOU TO READ THIS BOOK

If you believe that attitude is everything, and we do...

If you believe in the power of belief, and we do...

If you believe that your thoughts shape your reality, and we do...

If you believe that your emotional state profoundly affects your physiological wellbeing, and we do...

Then you will understand why we believe The Pickle Pledge was as important to our clinical outcomes as was all of the sophisticated medical technology and outstanding nursing care that we were blessed to receive during our hospital stays. Because of our commitment to The Pickle Pledge we are happier, healthier, more productive, and better off in virtually every dimension of our lives. If you make the commitment, you will be too.

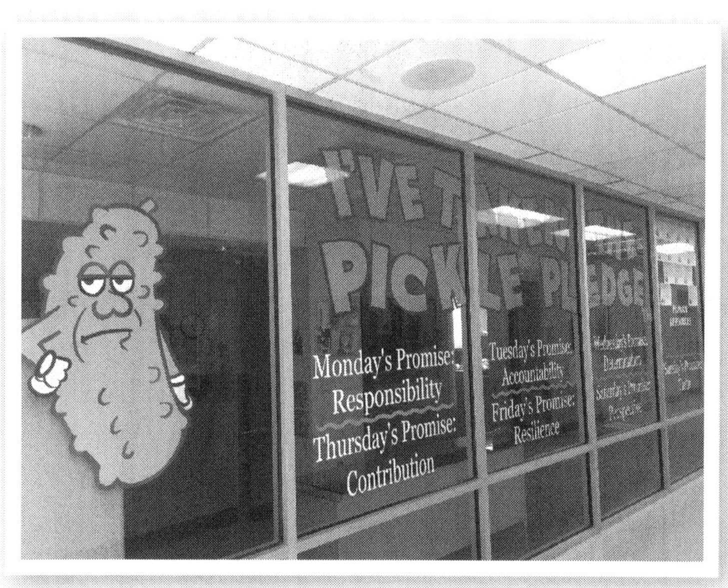
Monday's Promise:
Responsibility
Thursday's Promise:
Contribution
Tuesday's Promise:
Accountability
Friday's Promise:
Resilience

How the Book is Organized

This book is in six parts. Following the introductory section, Part 2 describes what we call "the healthcare crisis within" – the cost imposed on healthcare organizations by toxic emotional negativity. In Part 3 we shift the focus to the cost to the individual of working in a setting that is contaminated by toxic emotional negativity. Part 4 introduces The Pickle Pledge and shows you how you can use this simple promise to change your life in a profoundly positive way. Part 5 introduces The Pickle Challenge for Charity and shows you how you can foster a more positive and productive culture of ownership, and at the same time raise money for a worthwhile charity, one attitude at a time by turning complaints into contributions. Finally in Part 6 we wrap up with suggestions for next steps including a description of services provided by Values Coach.

PART 2
THE INNER HEALTHCARE CRISIS

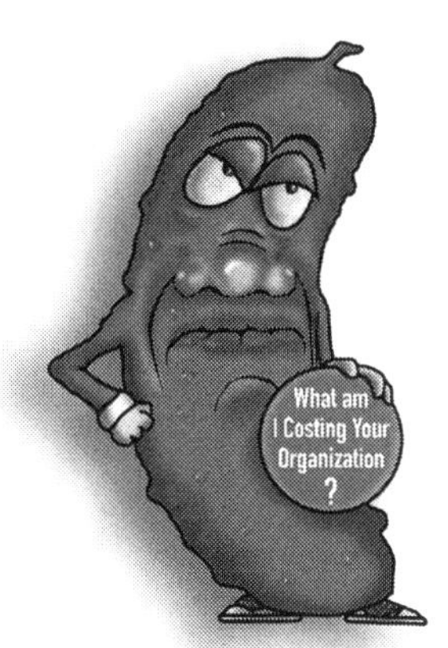

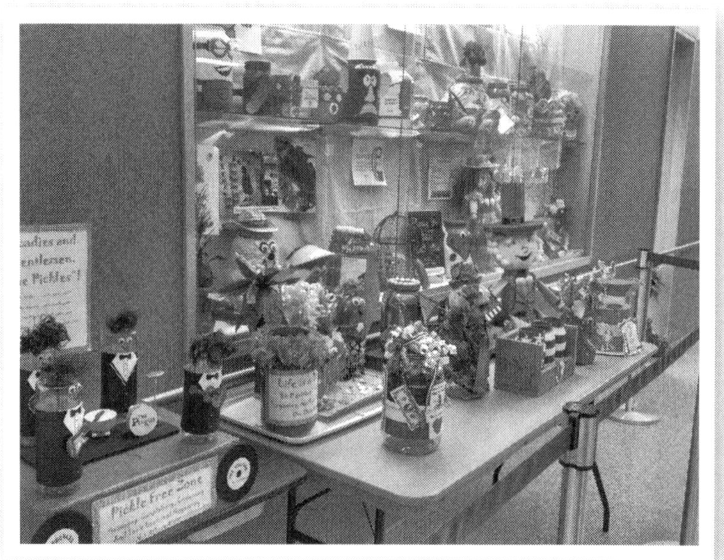

Turning Complaints into Contributions

The Organizational Cost of Toxic Emotional Negativity

For years we've seen headlines about the "healthcare crisis" related to cost, access, safety and quality. Many of these problems are largely, or completely, beyond the direct control of an individual hospital or even a large healthcare system. But there is another healthcare crisis. This one is on the inside and it is within our power to manage. This "crisis within" is reflected in the frequency with which terms such as bullying, lateral violence, incivility, passive-aggressiveness, disengagement, and other forms of toxic emotional negativity (TEN) show up in the healthcare literature. It is a leadership imperative to create a workplace environment in which such practices are not tolerated.

Gallup and other organizations that study employee engagement consistently find that, on average, only about 25 percent of employees are engaged, while 60 percent are not engaged and 15 percent are aggressively disengaged. There is obviously a huge variation between organizations, even within the same industry. The experience of being an employee or a customer of Costco vs. Walmart, Southwest Airlines vs. United Airlines, or Zappos vs. Payless Shoes could not be any more different, even though these companies recruit the same types of people to sell the same sorts of products to the same customer base. The difference is culture and the respective level of employee engagement or disengagement.

Unfortunately, despite the importance of the healing mission of healthcare organizations as opposed to, say, selling shoes, the problem of disengagement and toxic emotional negativity might be even greater in healthcare than in other industries. In the article "Where the Bullies Are" (*HR Magazine*, March 2016) Dana Wilkie writes that "bullying often occurs in workplaces where highly powerful people – or those with high-profile jobs – work alongside those with lower status," and identifies healthcare (along with education) as an industry where those conditions prevail. This becomes visibly reflected in negative attitudes and counterproductive behaviors in the healthcare workplace.

Values Coach conducts a Culture Assessment Survey that asks employees of client organizations to share their perceptions of that organization's culture. One of the most important questions asks people to assess, on a 5-point scale, the degree to which their coworkers "reflect positive attitudes, treat others with respect, and refrain from complaining, gossiping, or pointing fingers." In many organizations, more people disagree than agree with that statement, and almost nobody strongly agrees (see Chart 1).

Chart 1

Our people reflect positive attitudes, treat others with respect, and refrain from complaining, gossiping, or pointing fingers.

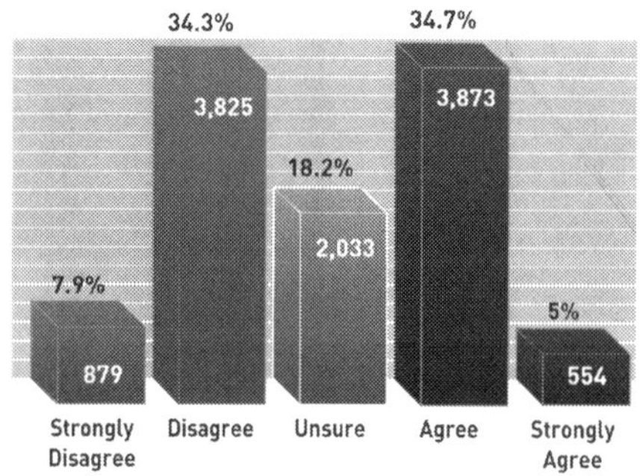

Total of 11,164 responses from 43 different hospitals and healthcare professional associations*

* Percentages do not total 100% due to rounding

Aggregated results from one of the questions in the Values Coach Culture Assessment Survey taken during 2015 and the first half of 2016

In his book *The Coming Jobs War*, Gallup CEO Jim Clifton estimates the cost to the U.S. economy of employee disengagement to be 500 billion dollars per year. Since healthcare accounts for nearly 20 percent of GDP, a straight extrapolation suggests that employee disengagement costs healthcare organizations close to 100 billion dollars per year. A recent research paper published by the Harvard Business Review ("It's Better to Avoid a Toxic Employee than Hire a Superstar") estimates that in the average organization the cost of emotional toxicity is more than $12,000 per year per employee.

The negative impact goes well beyond just the financial cost, though. It also registers in lowered patient satisfaction, employee disengagement, greater difficulty recruiting and retaining the best people, diminished image and reputation within the community, and increased risk of serious medical errors. In her *New York Times* magazine article "No Time to be Nice at Work" Georgetown University professor Christine Porath wrote that "people working in an environment characterized by incivility miss information that is right in front of them. They are no longer able to process it as well or as efficiently as they would otherwise." She cites a survey of more than 4,500 healthcare professionals in which "71 percent tied disruptive behavior, such as abusive, condescending or insulting personal conduct, to medical errors, and 27 percent tied such behavior to patient deaths."

In a poll of 800 managers and employees in 17 industries, Porath and Peterson reported that after exposure to incivility a substantial proportion of employees intentionally decreased time and effort spent at work, had reduced commitment to their organizations and to providing great service to customers, and 12% reported having left their jobs due to uncivil treatment.

The most pernicious reflection of TEN is bullying and lateral violence, the prevalence of which is reflected in book titles such as *Ending Nurse-to-Nurse Hostility*, *Toxic Nursing*, *When Nurses Hurt Nurses*, and *Do No Harm Applies to Nurses Too!*. A literature review by the authors revealed 115 articles with the word "bullying" in the title over the past five years – and that was just in the nursing literature. In the 2012 *American Nurse Today* article "Break the Bullying Cycle" Terri Townsend (citing original research from the University of Cincinnati) wrote: "Roughly 60 percent of new RNs quit their first job within 6 months of being bullied, and one in three new graduate nurses considers quitting nursing altogether because of abusive or humiliating encounters."

The situation was deemed sufficiently serious by the American Nurses Association that they issued a "Position Statement on Incivility, Bullying, and Workplace Violence" which states:

> Incivility can take the form of rude and discourteous actions, of gossiping and spreading rumors, and of refusing to assist a coworker. All of these are an affront to the dignity of the coworker and violate professional standards of respect. Such actions may also include name-calling, using a condescending tone, and expressing public criticism. The negative impact of incivility can be significant and far-reaching and can affect not only the targets themselves, but also bystanders, peers, stakeholders, and organizations. If left unaddressed, it may progress in some cases to threatening situations or violence.

Toxic emotional negativity is reflected in chronic complaining, gossip and rumor-mongering, passive-aggressive resistance to change, cynicism and pessimism, bullying and lateral violence. It exacts an enormous toll on employee morale, patient satisfaction, productivity, and virtually every other operating parameter. It is a leading contributor to stress and burnout, compassion fatigue, and costly unwanted turnover. Because emotions are contagious an emotionally negative healthcare workplace can actually cause iatrogenic emotional harm to patients in hospitals and residents in long-term care settings. We need to declare our hospitals, long-term care facilities, ambulatory clinics and other healthcare organizations to be Pickle-Free Zones. We owe it to caregivers and to the people they care for.

** This section adapted from the article "Creating a Positive Culture of Ownership" by Bob Dent and Joe Tye in the AONE publication Nurse Leader, June 2016*

Values Coach Culture Assessment Surveys at client organizations indicate that the cost of toxic emotional negativity and disengagement ranges from hundreds of thousands of dollars for a small critical access hospital to tens of millions of dollars for a larger medical center and hundreds of millions of dollars for a large healthcare system.

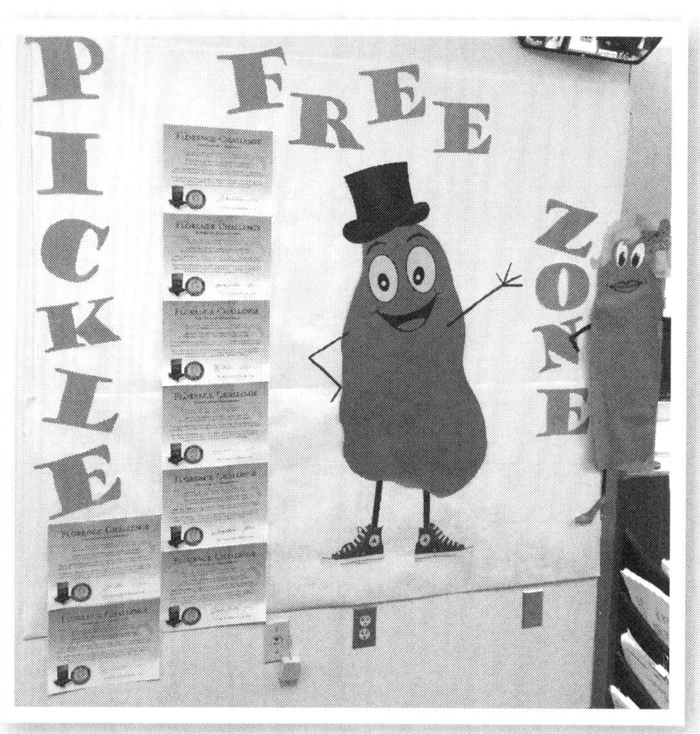
PICKLE
FREE
ZONE

AN OFTEN ABDICATED MANAGEMENT DUTY

There is an unfortunate level of learned helplessness on the part of healthcare leaders when it comes to dealing with the problem of toxic emotional negativity. One often hears comments like "that's just the way he/she is" in reference to bullying or toxically negative individuals, and "you can't change human nature" when it comes to eradicating toxic emotional negativity from the workplace. Quite to the contrary, toxic emotional negativity is not human nature; it is a choice one makes to inflict their bad attitude upon coworkers. As Joe wrote in *The Florence Prescription: From Accountability to Ownership*: "One toxically negative person can drag down the morale and the productivity of an entire work unit. It is a leadership responsibility to create a workplace where toxic emotional negativity is not tolerated."

One of the best predictors of a successful culture change initiative is enthusiastic engagement of the leadership team. This includes having the courage to raise the bar on expectations for positive attitudes and behaviors, constructively confronting those who refuse to meet those expectations, and having the determination and stamina to plow through resistance. When this happens people appreciate how wonderful it is to work in a place that is free from toxic emotional negativity and they become more intolerant of transgressors. Over time, just as no smoking policies are now enforced by cultural expectations and not by policing actions, "Pickle-Free Zones" begin to be enforced by the people who benefit from them.

> *"Whiners bring doom and gloom to the office. They aren't problem solvers; instead, they waste people's time with their tales of woe and expect others to solve their problems for them. They can be overly emotional and indecisive, and they may not act when they should."*
>
> Linda Swindling: *Stop Complainers and Energy Drainers: How to Negotiate Work Drama to Get More Done*

Managers' Responsibility for Protecting Their People from Toxic Emotional Negativity

It is a management duty to protect employees from the baleful influence to toxically negative coworkers. If someone comes to work wanting to work hard, to do a good job, to experience the joy of doing good work in a positive setting, and a manager allows bullies, emotional vampires and pickle-suckers to deprive that employee of these things, then that manager is failing at an important part of the job. Two of the questions in the Values Coach Culture Assessment Survey ask people to rate their organization on a 5-point scale from Strongly Agree to Strongly Disagree:

> Our managers effectively deal with toxic negative attitudes and behaviors in the workplace.
>
> Our people reflect positive attitudes, treat others with respect, and refrain from complaining, gossiping, or pointing fingers.

In almost every case, the shape of the response curves to these two questions is virtually identical. Quite clearly the ability of managers to effectively deal with toxic attitudes and behaviors determines the extent to which those attitudes and behaviors are tolerated.

When a manager fails to discipline a bully, or when a staff person listens to coworkers engaged in malicious gossip about another coworker behind that person's back without attempting to stop it, that lack of courage contributes to an unhealthy workplace culture where people's attitudes and behaviors are not compatible with the organization's stated values and cultural expectations.

Confronting the Wicked Witch of the Workplace

"Avoiding a toxic worker (or converting him to an average worker) enhances performance to a much greater extent than replacing an average worker with a superstar worker."

Michael Houseman and Dylan Minor: Toxic Workers
(Harvard Business School Working Paper 16-057)

Do you remember the Wicked Witch of the West from The Wizard of Oz? She is a perfect metaphor for the toxic employee in two ways. First, toxic employees prey upon positive people ("I'll get you my pretty" could be their mantra). They especially concentrate their venom on new employees in the attempt to suck them into their caustic emotional stew. This is why in healthcare one hears such things as "nurses eat their young" (a hideous metaphor if ever there was one!). It is a paramount responsibility of a manager to protect new people from the poisonous fangs of toxic emotional vampires.

Second, while they often seem to be popular and to have a clique of groupies hovering around them, in many cases those apparent hangers-on are just waiting and praying for that emotional vampire's manager to summon up the courage to deal with it. When that manager does finally discipline or discharge the emotional vampire, you'll hear people say "it's about time" – and perhaps even launch into a round of "Ding Dong the Witch is Dead" the way the Wicked Witch's soldiers did after Dorothy threw water on her.

In a blog posting (August 17, 2016) Seth Godin wrote that dysfunctional organizations are built slowly, one compromise at a time. Looking the other way at toxic emotional negativity because "we can't afford to lose that person" regardless of the emotional harm that he or she inflicts upon others is one of the most organizationally damaging of those compromises.

When the Manager is the Emotional Vampire

In January of 2015, Joe conducted a webinar for the American Nurses Association Leadership Institute on the subject of "Values-Based Leadership: Creating a Culture of Ownership." More than 3,000 individuals registered. Nearly 150 questions were submitted during the 15-minute Q&A session following the webinar. One of the most frequent, and most heartbreaking, questions was a variation of this: What if the emotional vampire (or the bully) is the boss? This is an example of one such question and Joe's response:

> *Question:* What can you do when the manager encourages negative attitudes by listening to complaints and listening to people talking about one another and does not put an effort in to stopping it and even most of the time joining in?
>
> *Response:* First let me make a comment about the duties and responsibilities of being a manager. Anyone who accepts the job title and the pay raise that goes with a management position gives up certain freedoms – including the freedom to act in a way that harms the organization. For a manager to condone, much less participate in, rumor-mongering, criticizing and

> complaining, and other forms of toxic emotional negativity is unethical. The organization is paying them to be a role model of leadership and oversee a positive workplace environment; it is unethical to accept that paycheck but then contribute to a more toxic workplace climate.

Many people who engage in toxic emotional negativity aren't even aware of the extent of their behavior, or of how harmful it is to the people around them. Sometimes simply calling their attention to it when they are gossiping or complaining – perhaps by asking them to put a quarter in your Pickle Jar – is all it will take to change their behavior. This is especially effective if a number of people on the unit are participating in the effort. But – and this is a very big but – you must do everything possible to make the confrontation light-hearted, soft-touch, and well-meaning. Something like this: "I believe the comment you just made might entitle you to make a donation to our unit's Pickle Jar." At the extreme, if a manager is bullying, intimidating, manipulating or otherwise engaging in behaviors that demean, degrade, or diminish individual employees then you and your colleagues will need the courage to take it to someone higher up on the organization chart or to Human Resources.

> *"Bullying damages the nursing profession. Bullying behavior not only is a direct violation of a nurse's code of ethics, but the mere existence of it tarnishes the reputation of the nursing profession. Bullying has a negative effect on the recruitment of new nurses while it puts current nurses, good nurses, at risk for leaving the profession, putting the entire profession of nursing in jeopardy."*
>
> Renee Thompson: *"Do No Harm" Applies to Nurses Too!: Strategies to Protect and Bully-proof Yourself at Work*

THE NON-NEGOTIABLE STARTING POINT FOR A POSITIVE WORKPLACE CULTURE

If you set out to create a healthy workplace, you could buy all the latest exercise equipment and set it up in an employee fitness center, offer broccoli and other nutritiously healthy foods in the cafeteria, give people paid time off for exercise and meditation and provide professional coaches to guide their exercise. But if you still allowed people to pollute the air with toxic cigarette smoke, you would not have a healthy workplace. Quite to the contrary. The non-negotiable first step to promoting a healthy environment is eradicating toxic influences such as ambient tobacco smoke.

It is the same with working to create a more positive culture of ownership. The essential first step is raising the level of intolerance for TEN. Just as one person lighting a cigarette instantly pollutes the lungs of everyone else in the room, one negative, bitter, cynical, sarcastic pickle-sucker can instantly pollute the emotional climate of a workplace, take the joy out of the work, poison relationships on the work unit, diminish the patient experience, and suck the energy out of any culture change initiative. Even worse, by dumping their TEN and negative attitudes on coworkers, they can diminish the quality of those coworkers' personal and professional lives and even imperil their health. As Daniel Goleman wrote in his book *Social Intelligence*, "When someone dumps their toxic feelings on us... they activate in us circuitry for those very same distressing emotions."

One 12-person clinical department in a mid-sized community hospital raised more than $80 during their Pickle Challenge week – meaning that more than 320 times during that week they caught themselves or each other BMW'ing. Prior to The Challenge, that department's patient satisfaction scores had consistently ranked in the bottom quartile; the next time scores came out they were in the top ten percent.

THE GOOD NEWS

There is good news on at least two fronts – personal and organizational. At the personal level, many of the behaviors of toxic emotional negativity (chronic complaining, talking about others behind their backs, and the like) are just bad habits that can be changed. We've heard many stories about people who, by getting clear about their own values and dreams, have made impressive attitude changes. We have seen how The Pickle Pledge can be life-changing. At the organization level, when a critical mass of people become aware of just how enervating and depressing it is to be subjected to toxic emotional negativity and make the commitment to personal change, a profound cultural transformation can occur.

Twenty years ago people smoked virtually everywhere and there was little that nonsmokers could do to protect themselves from being poisoned by the toxic smoke that permeated our environment. Today the situation has completely reversed and the smoking section is out by the garbage dumpster (or on most hospital campuses across the freeway). Having seen many successes over the past several years, including that at Midland Memorial Hospital, we are convinced that – using many of the same techniques – people can eradicate toxic emotional negativity from the workplace the way we, not all that long ago, eradicated toxic cigarette smoke. And we will all be a lot better off for having made the effort.

> *"The good news is that great and good people can leave an unhealthy workplace. It's also the bad news. It means that mediocre staff and management stay behind. Most sick environments don't want to take their own pulse and temp to see how they're doing; they are blinded to many of the behavior problems that create toxic workplaces."*
>
> Judith Briles: *Sabotage!: How to Deal with the Pit Bulls, Skunks, Snakes, Scorpions, & Slugs in the Healthcare Workplace*

Part 3
The Personal Cost of Toxic Emotional Negativity

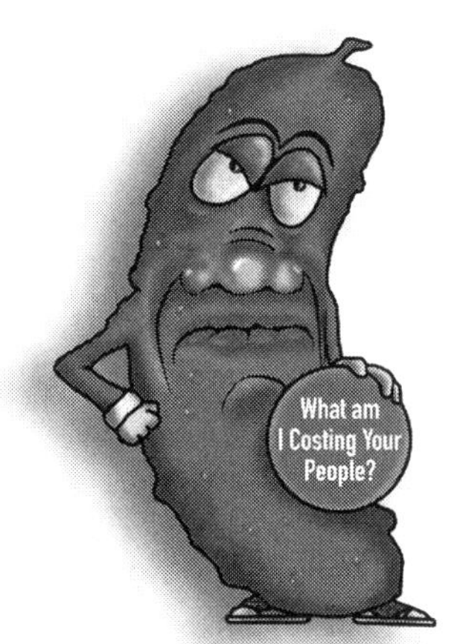

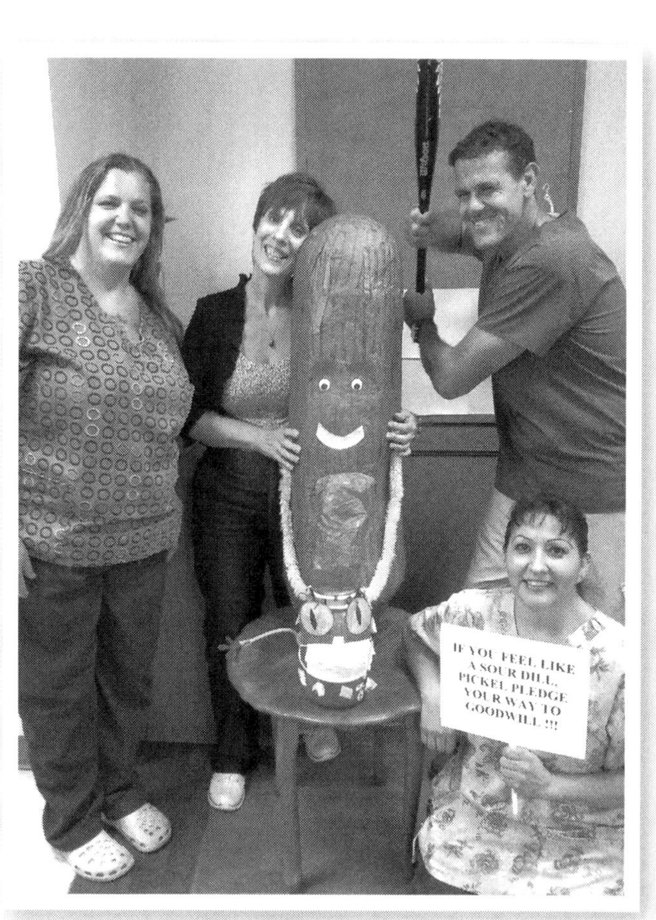
IF YOU FEEL LIKE
A SOUR DILL
PICKEL PLEDGE
YOUR WAY TO
GOODWILL !!!

Wasting Your Life One Complaint at a Time

"We complain to get sympathy, attention, and to avoid stepping up to something we're afraid of doing... We complain to get ourselves out of taking risks and doing things. The complaints seem legitimate, but they're thin excuses [for whining instead of doing]. Complaining is often a means of drawing attention to one's self."

Will Bowen: *A Complaint-Free World*

Your mind can only carry one thought at a time. You cannot multi-task thinking. Whenever you complain – whether you're saying it out loud or just thinking it – you block out all other thoughts. You cannot be thinking about the next steps you have to take on a project you're working on; you cannot be thinking about how much you love your family and appreciate the blessings in your life; and you cannot be thinking about how to be a stronger and better person.

The *I Ching* – a 3,000-year-old book of Chinese wisdom – tells us that every negative thought must be set aside before it takes root. Every negative thought is, one way or another, a form of complaining. With every negative, complaining thought, you put yourself in the role of "poor me" – the victim role. With every complaint, you are saying to yourself – and anyone else who happens to be listening – that the world is not doing enough to make your life more pleasant, convenient, and enjoyable. Complaining makes you weak and pathetic. Don't do it. You are better than that.

20 Ways that Complaining Diminishes Your Life

Think about the people you most admire. What quality or characteristic makes them worthy of admiration? Courage? Generosity? Humility? Confidence? Whatever you listed, we'll bet you anything you didn't include the fact that they complain a lot.

1. Complaining is malignant and contagious

Toxic emotional negativity is the emotional and spiritual equivalent of cigarette smoke. It is malignant and it is contagious. Attitudinal negativity of the type that is reflected in chronic complaining has been shown to be not just emotionally but physically harmful. It is toxic to heart and soul in the same way that cigarette smoke is damaging to the body. And just as one person lighting a cigarette will instantly pollute the lungs of everyone else in the room, one emotional vampire can suck the energy out of an entire roomful of otherwise positive and enthusiastic people.

2. Complaining is depressing

By its very nature complaining is being focused on bad stuff. Nobody complains about good things in their lives. And this focus on, and whining about, things that make you unhappy will make you even more unhappy.

3. Complaining is ingratitude

Think of complaining as the un-prayer. Instead of expressing thankfulness for the blessings of your life, complaining is saying that – despite all that you might have been blessed with – it's not enough. The world has not bent over backwards to make your life sufficiently comfortable, convenient, and enjoyable. So you complain. You cannot simultaneously be thankful for what you do have and resentful for what you don't have but think you are entitled to. Most people living in the western world (and in most of the rest of the world for that matter) have more to be grateful for than they have to be resentful about. Make sure that gratitude shines through in your attitudes and in your actions instead of letting resentment show through in whining and complaining.

4. Complaining is an excuse for laziness, avoidance, and procrastination

Complaining is faux action. It's a great excuse for avoiding problems and the work that's required to fix them. Complaining about something makes you feel like you're doing something about a problem without actually having to do something about it. It's easier to complain about potholes in the street than it is to show up at a city council meeting with a petition signed by a hundred people. It's easier to complain about how underpaid you are, or how much of your paycheck goes to taxes, than it is to work overtime or learn new skills to increase your income.

5. Complaining is an excuse for cowardice

It's easier to complain about another person behind his or her back than it is to confront that person about the attitudes or behaviors you are complaining about. It's also the coward's way out. And by complaining instead of having the courage to act, you assure that the situation will endure and inevitably get worse.

6. Complaining is Resistance

In his book *The War of Art,* Steven Pressfield describes Resistance (he capitalizes the word the way an historian would capitalize Black Death or Great Depression) as the inner barrier that prevents people from being authentic and doing their most creative work. Complaining is a manifestation of Resistance. It's a lot easier to sit at the airport terminal complaining about the one-hour delay in your flight than it is to use that unexpectedly free hour to write the next page in your Great American Novel.

> *"A victim act is a form of passive aggression. It seeks to achieve gratification not by honest work or a contribution made out of one's experience or insight or love, but by the manipulation of others through silent (and not-so-silent) threat... Casting yourself as a victim is the antithesis of doing your work. Don't do it. If you're doing it, stop."*
>
> Steven Pressfield: *The War of Art: Break through the Blocks and Win Your Inner Creative Battles*

7. Complaining keeps you stuck in the past

We love to hang on to our drama-trauma, which is what you are doing every time you complain. You are living in the past. Even if you're complaining about something that you think might happen in the future, the reason for that bleak outlook is always a projection of things that have happened in the past. That sad past is a trap. A coyote that has its foot caught in a trap will gnaw it off. It's willing to go through short-term pain and long-term limitation in order to gain its freedom. Any time you catch yourself whining and complaining, remember this: *It's better to be a 3-legged coyote than a 4-legged fur coat!*

8. Complaining is an outward projection of negative self-talk

The words that come out of your mouth are an outward projection of what is going on between your ears. In a very real sense it is an echo. When you complain you are not only complaining to the listeners outside of your body – you are also telling the listener on the inside of your body that at this moment your world sucks. Your subconscious mind takes whatever you say as gospel truth, so whenever you complain you diminish the self-esteem, self-confidence and self-worth of that inner child.

> *"Speaking wisely is essential when you speak to yourself… Words matter. We cannot risk speaking untruths to ourselves because of the strong likelihood that we will believe them"*
>
> Jennifer Rothschild: *Self Talk, Soul Talk: What to Say When You Talk to Yourself*

9. Complaining is an energy suck

You only have so much energy in a day – and chances are that most days you wish you'd had more. Complaining drains your precious life energy with absolutely zero positive results to show for it. But you don't need to take our word for it. The next time you catch yourself complaining about something check in with your energy level. If you're being honest with yourself, you will recognize that it's been depleted.

10. Complaining is an insidious form of gossip

Complaining about another person, especially when that individual is not present to hear it, is almost always damaging to that person's reputation. By definition, you don't complain about how much you like another person or how much you admire their strength of character and the work they do. You complain about the things you don't like about them, creating a negative impression of that person in the minds of listeners. Complaining about another person is a form of trash talk, and as Cheryl Dellasega & Rebecca L. Volpe note in their book *Toxic Nursing: Managing Bullying, Bad Attitudes, and Total Turmoil*, "Gossip and negative trash talk can take on a life of their own, poisoning a unit and spilling into other venues such as home and leisure activities."

11. COMPLAINING IS AN INSIDIOUS FORM OF BULLYING

When someone is prevented from being positive, enthusiastic and productive in their work because of the chronic complaining of one or more coworkers, that is a subtle and insidious form of bullying. It takes courage to resist the peer pressure sucking you into the emotional swamp created by chronic complainers, much less to confront these people about their toxic negative attitude. And in that respect, it feels remarkably similar to being emotionally abused in more overt ways. This is especially true when the chronic complainer has a domineering personality, which is often how emotional vampires come across.

> *"For some, the painful impact from the stress of incivility remains for years and, in some cases, results in diagnosable mental illnesses."*
>
> Cynthia Clark: *Creating & Sustaining Civility in Nursing Education*

12. COMPLAINING IS FINGER-POINTING

Complaining is almost never directed at the person doing the complaining. It is a way of avoiding personal responsibility by pointing a finger somewhere else. The person who complains about a coworker not pulling his or her load rarely looks in the mirror to honestly ask if the same couldn't be said about their own performance.

13. COMPLAINING MAKES YOU BORING – AND BORED

In his book *And Never Stop Dancing* Dr. Gordon Livingston writes that complainers bore the people who have to listen to them, and eventually bore themselves with their tales of misery and unhappiness. As Lou Holtz put it in his book *Winning Every Day*, "Remember, if you have a problem, it's your problem. Solve it. Don't blame other people. Don't burden people with your complaints. Ninety percent of the people you meet don't care about your troubles. The other 10 percent are glad you have them."

14. COMPLAINING IS HOLDING ON TO A GRUDGE

You wouldn't complain if you didn't feel aggrieved about something, and often that something is related to what another person has done. Perhaps without being aware of it, you are carrying a grudge. There's an old saying that holding a grudge is like drinking poison in hopes of hurting someone else. Any time you complain about another person, that is exactly what you are doing.

15. COMPLAINING IS PARENTING MALPRACTICE

One of the worst things a parent can do to a child is to teach him or her that work sucks. If a child listens to Mom or Dad talking about how important it is for them to get a job, then hears Mom/Dad complaining about how miserable their own job is, how excited do you think that child will be about the prospect of going to work? Complaining parents run the risk of raising their kids as Junior Dilberts who have their own negative attitudes about the world of work. And those kids will go out into the world and compete for jobs with other kids who've been taught that work should matter, and that they should be passionate about that work. And those kids who've been taught that work sucks run the risk of ending up dead-ended in dead-end jobs.

> *"Work is love made visible. And if you cannot work with love but only with distaste, it is better that you should leave your work and sit at the gate of the temple and take alms of those who work with joy."*
>
> Kahlil Gibran: *The Prophet*

16. Complaining crowds out compassion

Much has been written about compassion fatigue in healthcare. It is a real and serious problem and should be treated as such. However (here comes the tough love message), there is also a very real danger of chronic complaining making compassion fatigue worse. Because it saps energy and kills enthusiasm, complaining about the work or the patients can accelerate the symptoms of compassion fatigue – which in turn gives more reason to complain – sparking a "circling the drain" sort of emotional downward spiral.

17. Complaining fosters pessimism

You complain because of the feeling that things aren't right – something is making you unhappy or you wouldn't be complaining. If you're unhappy with your situation today but don't do anything other than complain about it, what reason could there possibly be for you to think that things will be any better in the future? The more you complain about your present, the more pessimistic you are going to be about your future. One definition of insanity is that it's doing the same things over and over and expecting a different outcome. By that definition, what would you call complaining about a problem without actually doing anything to fix it?

> *"It is totally normal to focus on how you are screwing up; unfortunately, by doing so, you make it more likely that you will screw up even more in the future."*
>
> Jason Selk and Tom Bartow (with Matthew Rudy): *Organize Tomorrow Today: 8 Ways to Retrain Your Mind to Optimize Performance at Work and in Life*

18. Complaining is the ultimate waste of time

Don't just take our word for this one – listen to someone who truly knows what he's talking about. Randy Pausch knew he was dying of pancreatic cancer when he wrote the book *The Last Lecture* (with Jeffrey Zaslow). He appreciated the preciousness of every second when he wrote: "Complaining does not work as a strategy. We all have finite time and energy. Any time we spend whining is unlikely to help us achieve our goals. And it won't make us happier." If you'd put one-tenth the energy you waste on complaining on actually trying to solve the problem you're whining about, he wrote, "you'd be surprised how well things can work out." Instead of complaining about the fact that he was going to die much too young and not be able to see his young children grow up, he wrote a book that was a letter to the people they would one day become – a book that has touched the lives of millions of others as well. Including the two of us.

19. Complaining takes years off your life

There is evidence that toxic emotional negativity, as reflected in chronic complaining, is bad for your health and can reduce your lifespan, but that's not what we're talking about here. We're talking about the minutes, hours, days and ultimately years of your life that are wasted on complaining. Because the human mind can only carry one thought at a time, when you are complaining your mind cannot focus on anything else. You cannot simultaneously be complaining and be thinking about how much you love your family, what more you can do in your work, the book you want to write or the business you want to start, or anything else. Those precious moments of your life are gone – poof! – up in the smoke of one complaint after another.

20. Complaining is Taking Up Residence in the Valley of the Shadow

The 23rd Psalm does not say "Yea, though I take up permanent residence in the valley of the shadow of death," it says "though I *walk through* the valley of the shadow of death." To be sure, some people have chosen to set up a tent, or move into a condo, in that dark and dreary valley. They whine and complain and never enjoy the sunshine of love or life. But make no mistake – they have made a choice to live in the shadows rather than to keep walking toward the light.

One workshop participant told Joe that if it weren't for complaining, she would never speak with her mother, who lived with her. But she agreed to enlist the two of them for The Pickle Challenge. Several months later, Joe heard from her. At first, she said, the house had been very quiet. But after a while she and her mother – for the first time in her life – began speaking about things that really mattered instead of just going back and forth on the complaints of the day. It was, she said, a miracle.

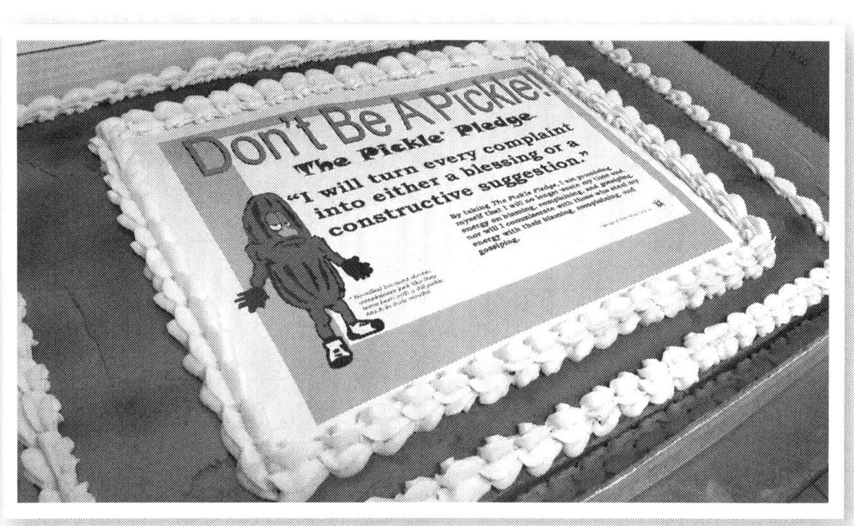

Don't Be A Pickle!
The Pickle* Pledge
"I will turn every complaint into either a blessing or a constructive suggestion."

You Have to Be Willing to Be Weird

Imagine you show up at the airport to catch a flight and there are only two people in the waiting area. And one of them is really weird. The first person is slouched down in the chair with a giant cinnamon roll on one knee and a latte overflowing with whipped cream on the other, reading the sports page of *USA Today*. The other is over by the window doing pushups. In our society, which one of those two would be considered weird? And what is wrong with this picture?

That is a great metaphor for the challenge of being a positive Spark Plug sort of person where you work. If you are the person who, metaphorically speaking, does pushups by the window, the emotional vampires will call you all sorts of nasty names, usually behind your back. Names like Pollyanna, overachiever, quota-buster, apple-polisher, brownnoser, suck-up, and the like. Think of how many ways we've learned to tell someone else to sit down, shut up, put a basket over their candle and be mediocre, beginning with being called teacher's pet in kindergarten. The Pickle Pledge is a form of rebellion against those toxic negative expectations and a commitment to do your pushups, even if the emotional vampires ridicule you for doing them.

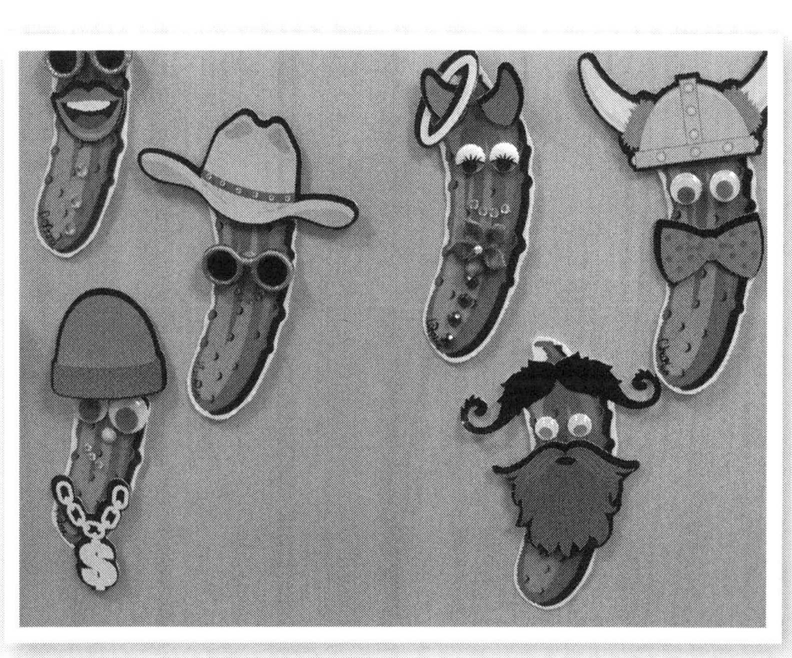

WHAT MADE "THE GREATEST GENERATION" GREAT

In his book *With the Old Breed* about his combat experiences as a Marine during the Pacific campaigns of World War II, E.B. Sledge wrote about how disappointing it was for soldiers to return from the unbelievable hardships and dangers they had experienced while fighting for their country and be confronted with people "who griped because America wasn't perfect, or their coffee wasn't hot enough, or they had to stand in line and wait for a train or bus [and other] trivial inconveniences."

The greatest generation described by Tom Brokaw in his book of that title survived the hardships of the Great Depression and the horrors of World War II and went on to shape the most secure, affluent, and comfortable society the world has ever known – the society of which we are all beneficiaries. What if, instead of rolling up their sleeves and going to work, they'd sat around complaining about how hard their lives had been? Where would we be today?

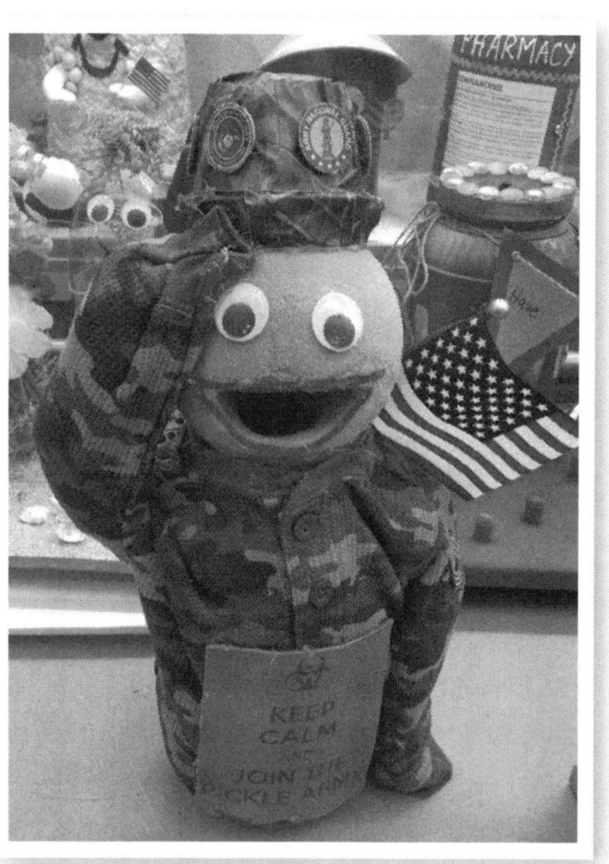
PHARMACY
KEEP
CALM

A GREAT DEFINITION OF A GREAT PLACE TO WORK

Fortune magazine uses a sophisticated assessment methodology to select the 100 Best Places to Work in America. One of the most insightful comments in the 2016 edition was from Stanley Bing, who writes the always humorous and usually cynical article "While You Were Out" on the magazine's last page (it's sort of like Dilbert with an intellect). In an article called "Making a Workplace Great" Bing wrote:

> A company is a great place to work if you can wake up every morning and go to the office or plant or cubicle farm with a spring in your step and a good, solid feeling that you're not wasting the one life God gave you doing somebody else's business and none of your own.

It's easy to overlook the most important point in this prescription: No organization ever hires anyone for any reason other than to do its business. It doesn't matter whether it's General Motors, Google, or the church on the corner. No matter what industry it's in, no matter whether it's for profit or not for profit, no matter how hard it works to be a great place to work, unless your name is over the door no organization will ever hire you and pay you to do your own business.

So while General Motors or Google or the church on the corner can go out of its way to make your work life pleasant, whether or not they are meeting Stanley Bing's definition of a great place to work is up to you, not them. If you are thinking like an owner and a partner and making the business of the organization your business as well, then you can make it a great place to work. On the other hand, if your attitude is "another day, another dollar – work sucks then you die" it does not matter what the employer does, because you are, in Bing's words, wasting the one life that God has given you doing somebody else's business because you have not taken ownership for the work itself. You have not made the business of the organization your business as well – Bing's definition of a great place to work.

Problems and Predicaments

A problem has a solution. A predicament does not have a solution.

If your local city council can fix it, you have a problem. If it takes an act of Congress, you have a predicament.

If you have a problem, deal with it. If you have a predicament, live with it. Either way, don't waste your precious life's energy whining about it.

One more thing: some predicaments can, over time, be transformed into problems and eventually solved, but it takes determination, hard work and sustained perseverance. Complaining about a predicament never turned it into a solvable problem.

If you can learn how to turn your problems into questions, you are better equipped to find a solution. It's how you go about finding solutions to the problems. If it's related to nursing practice, look for best practices or evidence to improve. If it's related to the workplace environment, work with your colleagues in a professional governance setting to improve. The fact is that we all own this together.

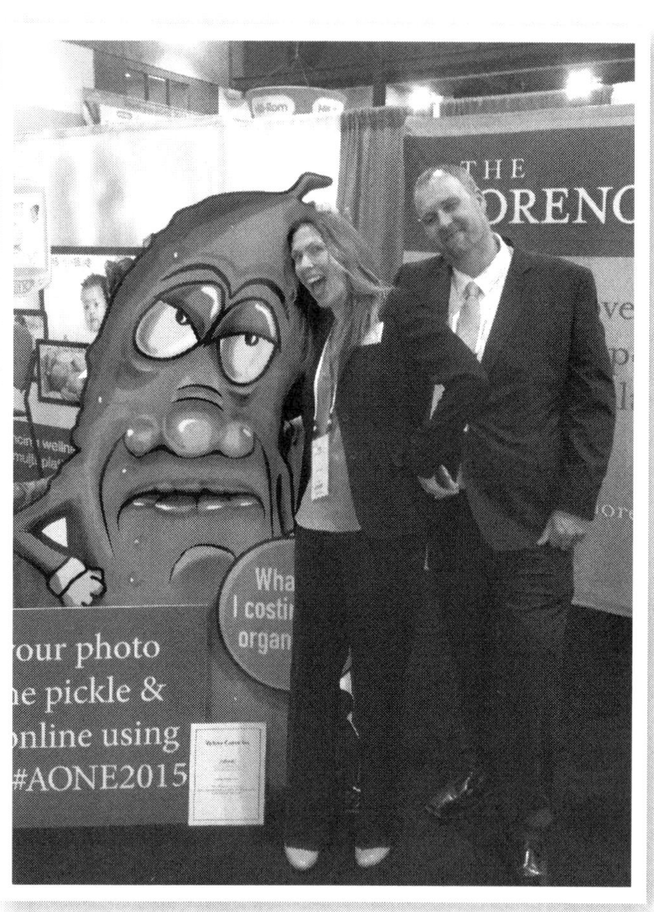
THE
#AONE2015

VENTING CAN BE TOXIC AND ABUSIVE

It's often said that "venting" is a legitimate form of complaining – usually by people who consider it a God-given right to dump their negative thoughts and emotions on innocent bystanders, often without warning them of what's about to happen. Nothing could be further from the truth. Here are definitions of the word "venting" from The Free Dictionary:

> Forceful expression or release of pent-up thoughts or feelings: *give vent to one's anger.*
>
> An opening permitting the escape of fumes, a liquid, a gas, or steam.
>
> The small hole at the breech of a gun through which the charge is ignited.
>
> The excretory opening of the digestive tract in animals such as birds, reptiles, amphibians, and fish.

As a metaphor, the word "venting" is perfect for what you are doing to the person upon whom you are venting. You are releasing noxious fumes, firing a deadly charge, dumping upon that hapless victim your own emotional poop. And while you might feel better once you're done dumping your emotional poop on someone else, it is almost certain that the person being dumped upon will feel worse. If you feel the need to vent, there are people who get paid to listen and who are trained to help. Go to a professional – don't contaminate family, friends and coworkers with your emotional poop.

One employee at a hospital that had taken The Pickle Challenge for Charity was going through a particularly difficult time at home, and she was severely depressed. One day, while reciting The Pickle Pledge in her department's daily huddle, she realized that a big part of her problem was participating in the BMW Club. Simply mentioning her troubles seemed to spark a shark feed of complaining: "You think *that's* bad – you should see what I have to put up with." She said she learned to tell the difference between a true friend and a bitch buddy, and when she started spending more time with the former and less time with the latter her life began to get a whole lot better.

Bring The Pickle Challenge home to your family

Every time either of us speaks to a group about The Pickle Pledge and The Pickle Challenge for Charity, we have someone come up afterward and ask if we can come home with them and "fix" a spouse or adolescent child (we also get lots of suggestions that we go to Washington D.C. and "fix" the politicians who work there). Of course, we cannot "fix" anyone, including members of your family. But if you will take The Pickle Challenge home and with a firm but loving hand invite your family members to join you in depositing quarters in a decorated pickle jar every time they began to complain about or blame other people for their problems, you will be amazed at the results. As a side benefit, that pickle jar full of quarters might become the down payment for that Caribbean cruise you've been dreaming of.

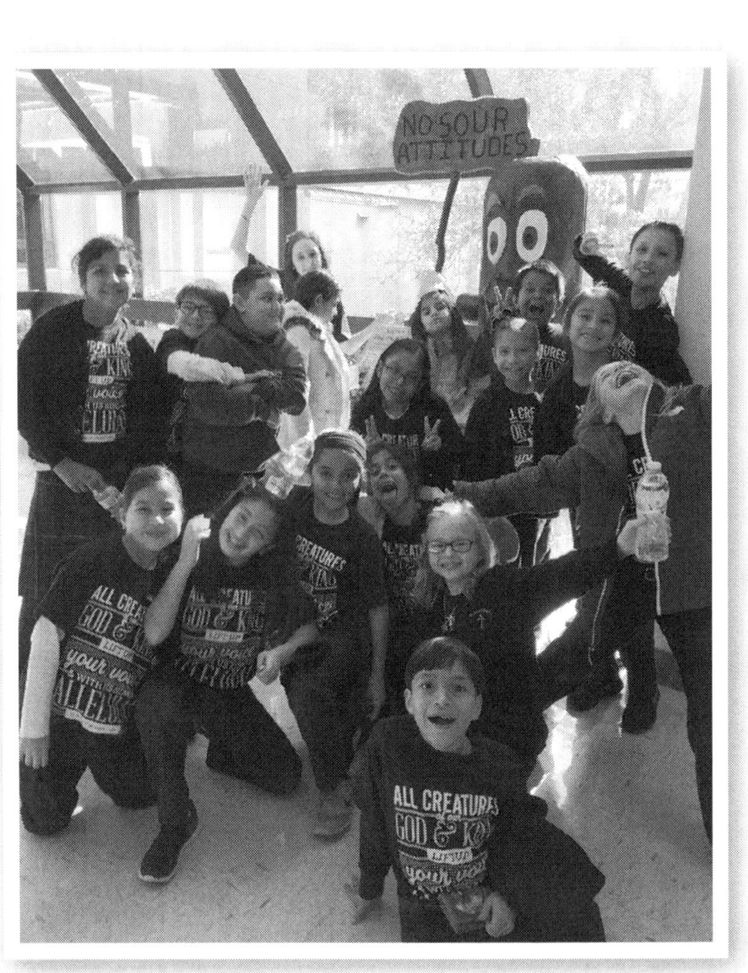
NO SOUR
ATTITUDES
ALL CREATURES

STAY OUT OF THE VICTIM SPIRAL

You can be a victim living in the past or you can be a visionary focused on the future, but you cannot be in both time zones at once. Every time you complain you fall into the victim spiral:

Complaining → Learned Helplessness → Blame Game → Victim Syndrome

When you complain about something you are implicitly saying that there's nothing you can do about it – otherwise you would be working to fix the problem instead of just whining about it. And since you've decided that you're helpless to do anything about it – learned helplessness – it must be someone else's fault so you find blame in another quarter. And as soon as you adopt the position that you are unhappy about something that is beyond your control because of someone else, you become, in your own mind, a victim. Don't do it.

At one VA medical center, a counselor working with a PTSD support group shared The Pickle Pledge with the group. She later heard from several of the men in the group that it had become an important part of their therapy. As one veteran put it, making that promise helped him to stop seeing himself as the victim of things that had happened in the past – and that would never un-happen – and to start focusing on the things that he still could do in the future.

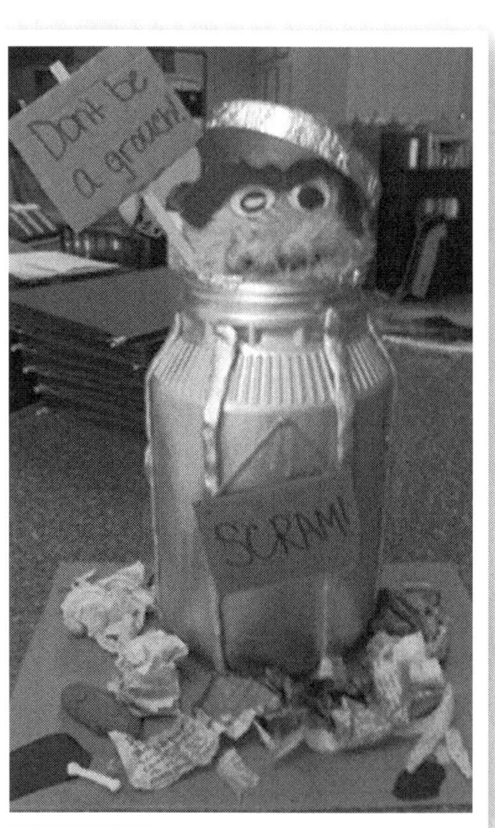
Don't be a grouch!
SCRAM!

MAKE A COMMITMENT – TO YOURSELF, YOUR COWORKERS, AND THE PEOPLE YOU SERVE

A culture of ownership is characterized by people who are emotionally positive, self empowered, and fully engaged. When you make that commitment yourself you will be happier and more productive; when everyone in your work unit makes that commitment you will do a better job of serving your patients and residents and of supporting one another. You can download The Florence Challenge Certificate of Commitment at www.TheFlorenceChallenge.com. Ask everyone in your department or unit to sign it and post them in a visible manner as an ongoing reminder of the type of people you want to be and the sort of organization in which you want to work.

THE

FLORENCE CHALLENGE

Certificate of Commitment

BY TAKING THE FLORENCE CHALLENGE I AM COMMITTING TO MYSELF, MY COWORKERS, AND THE PATIENTS WE SERVE TO BE:

EMOTIONALLY POSITIVE by taking to heart The Pickle Pledge and turning every complaint into either a blessing or a constructive suggestion.

SELF EMPOWERED by taking to heart the 7 promises of The Self-Empowerment Pledge: Responsibility, Accountability, Determination, Contribution, Resilience, Perspective, and Faith.

FULLY ENGAGED by being committed, engaged, and passionate in my work; taking initiative and being an effective steward of resources; fostering a spirit of belonging and fellowship; and taking pride in my work, my profession, my organization, and myself.

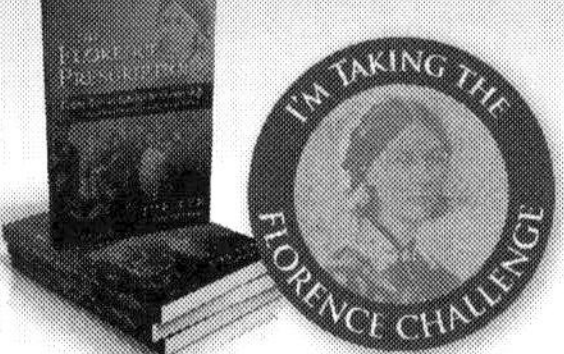

Signature Date

TheFlorenceChallenge.com

You can download and print The Florence Challenge Certificate of Commitment for everyone where you work at the Resources page of: www.TheFlorenceChallenge.com

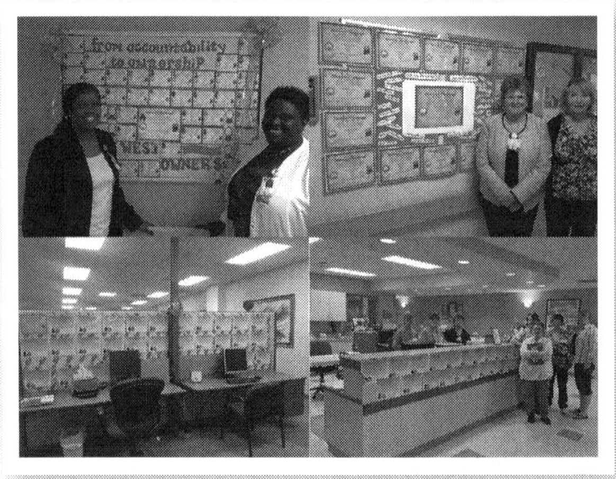

Part 4
The Pickle Pledge

I've Taken The Pickle Pledge

"I will turn every complaint into either a blessing or constructive suggestion."

By taking **The Pickle Pledge**, I am promising myself that I will no longer waste my time and energy on blaming, complaining, and gossiping, nor will I commiserate with those who steal my energy with their blaming, complaining, and gossiping.

ValuesCoach.com • TheFlorenceChallenge.com

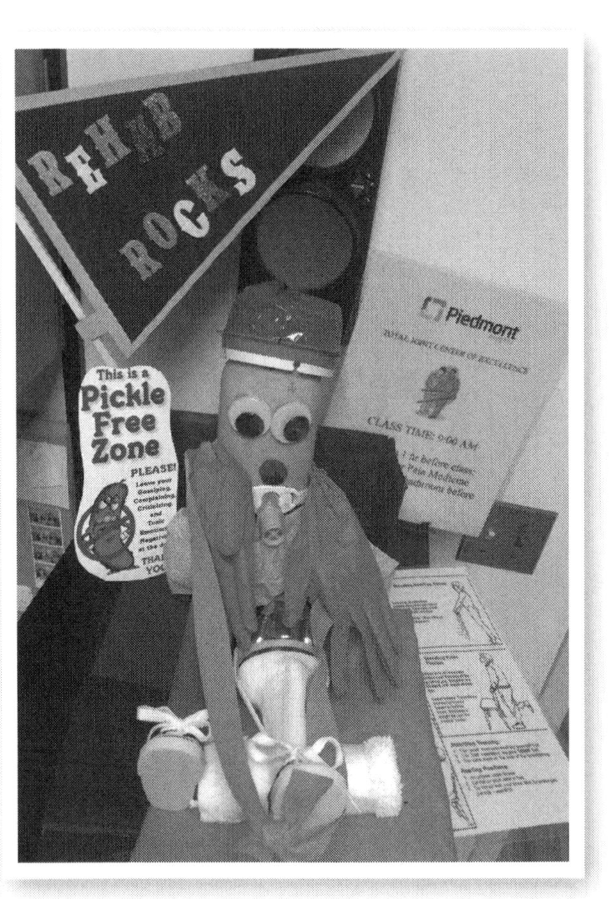
REHAB
ROCKS
This is a
Pickle
Free
Zone
PLEASE!
Piedmont
CLASS TIME: 9:00 AM

The Promise that Will Change Your Life

If there was a simple promise that would make you happier, more productive, more resilient, more likeable, and a better person in every other dimension, would you make that promise to yourself and then do your best to try and keep it?

There is such a promise: The Pickle Pledge. It's simple but not always easy. At least not at first. But if you keep making this promise to yourself you will find that you no longer allow little problems and minor inconveniences to bother you; you will find yourself looking for the best in other people and in every situation; you will discover that you have more positive emotional energy and a brighter outlook on your day; and you will discover that other people react to you in a more positive and friendly manner.

You might also find that some of the people who you used to hang around the water cooler with complaining, commiserating, and gossiping are not happy with this new you. Remember what we said about the difference between true friends and bitch buddies – and that you want more of the former and none of the latter.

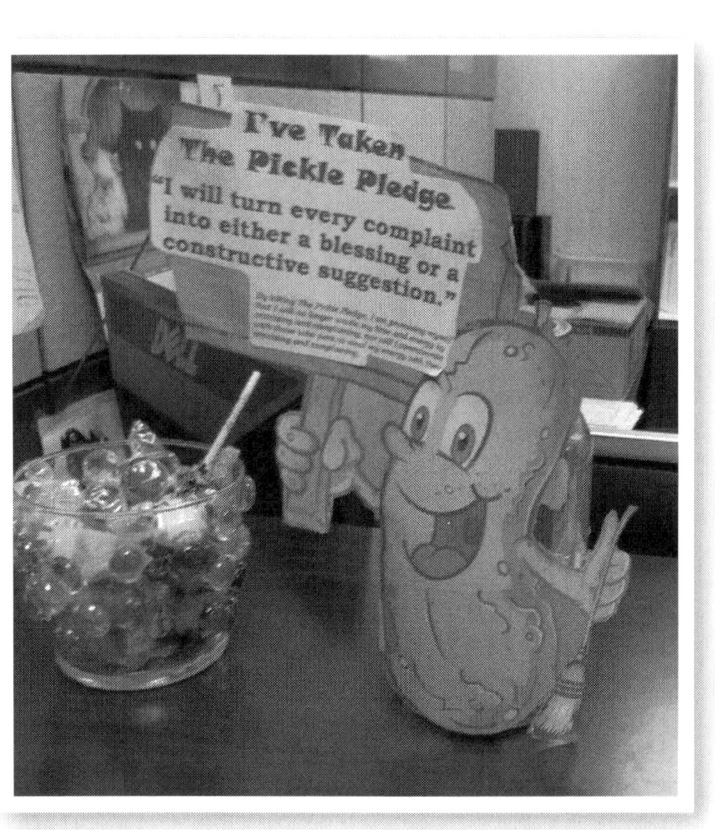
I've Taken
The Pickle Pledge.
"I will turn every complaint
into either a blessing or a
constructive suggestion."

Turning complaints into blessings and constructive suggestions

There really is nothing you can complain about that cannot instead be turned into a blessing and/or a constructive suggestion. Got a headache? Thank God for modern pharmacology – there's a pill for that (the blessing). And drink a glass of water, because the first symptom of dehydration is a headache (the constructive suggestion). Had to park six blocks away and walk all the way in to the mall? Thank God you have legs and money to spend in the mall, and that you don't live in Somalia where a mall is an unheard of luxury (the blessing). And if you would eat fewer donuts and spend a bit more time at the gym, maybe walking six blocks wouldn't have been such a hardship (the constructive suggestion).

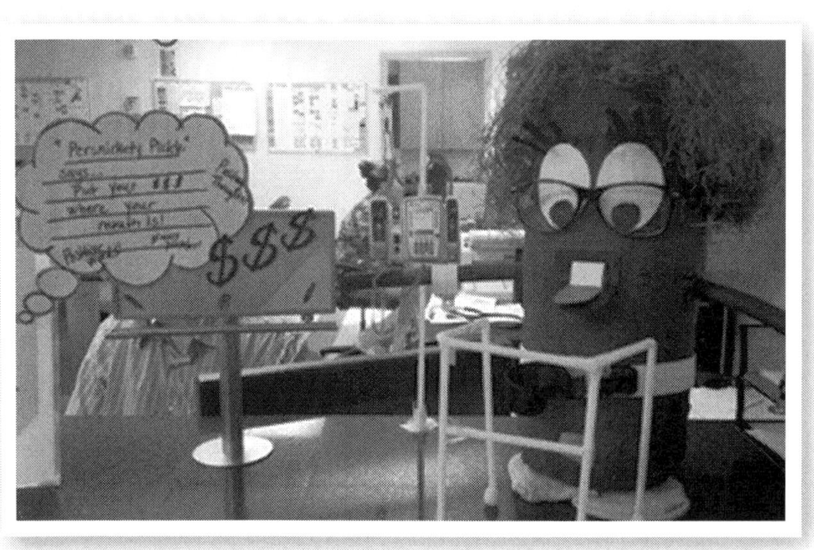
"Persnickety Patty"
says...
Put your $$$
where your
mouth is!
$$$

THE FOOTNOTE – CHANGING YOUR REFERENCE GROUP

You are subtly but profoundly influenced by the people you spend time with and identify with – what sociologists call your reference group. That can be a good thing when it comes to professional associations, service clubs and the like. But if you spend much time with people who are chronically complaining about, and blaming other people for, their problems, then their toxic attitudes will inevitably begin to rub off on you. You might not be aware of it when it's happening, might not admit the possibility that you can be subject to such peer pressure, but you cannot prevent it from happening. That's why the footnote to The Pickle Pledge is so important. It says: *By taking The Pickle Pledge I am promising myself that I will no longer waste my time and energy on blaming, complaining, and gossiping, nor will I commiserate with those who steal my energy with their blaming, complaining, and gossiping.* Toxic emotional negativity is a disease against which you must inoculate yourself; pickle-suckers and emotional vampires are the vectors that transmit that disease against which you must protect yourself.

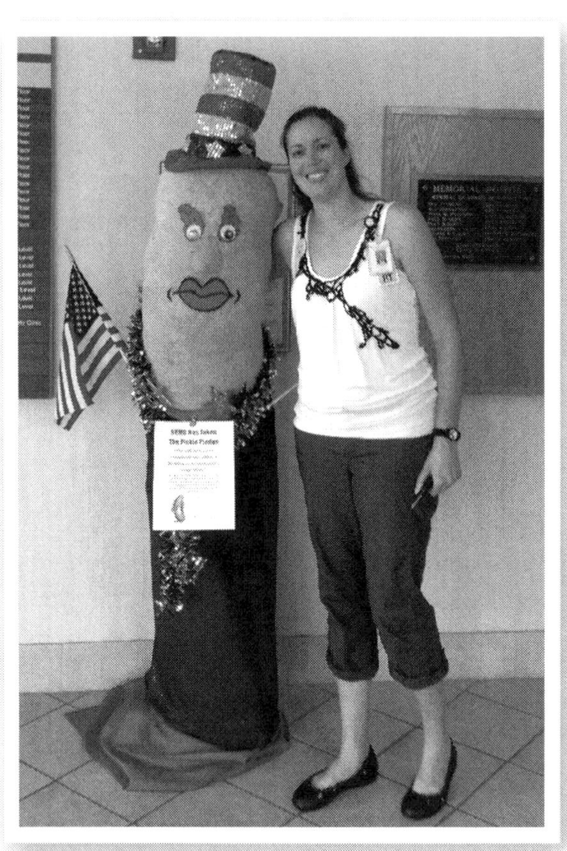
The Pickle Pledge

MAKE YOUR WORKPLACE, AND YOUR HOME, A PICKLE-FREE ZONE

Toxic emotional negativity – as reflected in chronic complaining, gossiping, and bullying behaviors – is the emotional and spiritual equivalent of cigarette smoke in the air. In its own way it is just as malignant. And just as we once had to declare our workspaces, and our homes, to be smoke-free zones to protect our health from inconsiderate smokers, today we can declare Pickle-Free Zones to protect ourselves (and our families at home) from inconsiderate Pickle-Suckers. Today we no longer need to post no-smoking signs in public places because of the profound ways in which public acceptance of smoking have changed. Imagine how much better our organizations – and our world – would be if we could do the same with toxic emotional negativity!

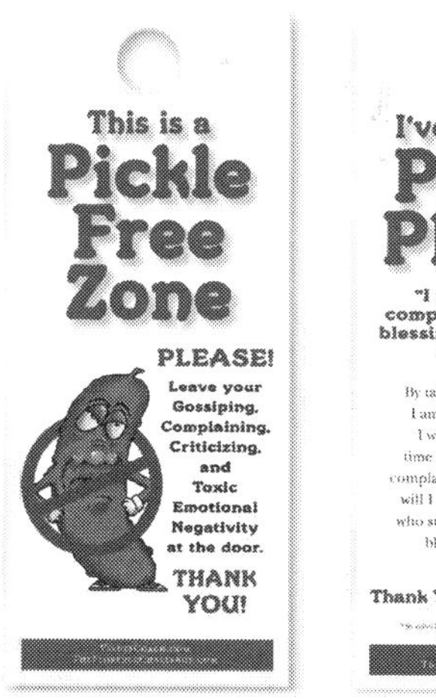

Pickle-Free Zone posters and door hangers are available at The Pickle Challenge website.

At Midland Memorial Hospital leaders from around the organization gather in the main lobby to recite the Pickle Pledge and the daily promise from The Self Empowerment Pledge every morning at 8:16 sharp. One morning a school teacher from a small town more than 50 miles away walked by as the Pickle Pledge was being recited. Soon after, she googled "The Pickle Pledge" and sent the information to the principal of the school. She called back to tell us how much it meant to her, and that they were going to start reciting The Pickle Pledge at her school each day.

---

10 Ways The Pickle Pledge Will Make You a Better Person

1. You will be more optimistic

When you complain about the things that are making you unhappy now you subconsciously set yourself up for more future disappointment and failure. But when you seek the blessing and the constructive suggestion in every obstacle or setback, you learn to see opportunities instead of barriers, doors instead of walls.

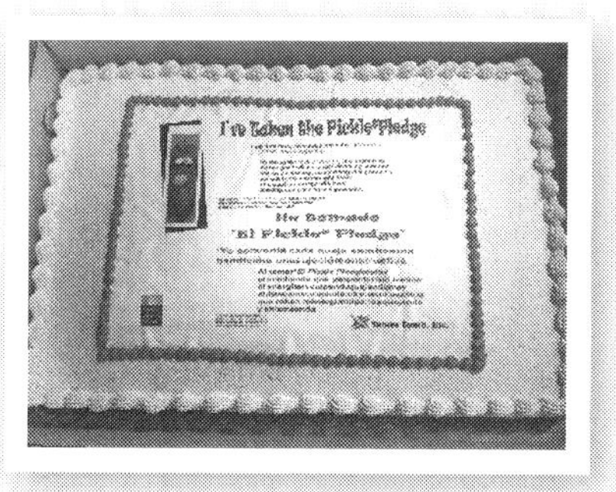

When Joe conducts his Spark Your Dream Workshop he gives participants a t-shirt. On the front the shirt is blank so they can draw a picture of their dream. On the back it says: *Define your future by your hopes and not by your fears, by your dreams and not by your memories.*

2. YOU WILL BE MORE COURAGEOUS

Complaining reflects a failure of courage. There is a lot less risk involved in complaining about something than there is in actually doing something about it. *Fear is a reaction, courage is a decision.* When you commit to The Pickle Pledge you will find that you have more courage to deal with problems rather than just complaining about them, and to persevere toward a solution even though the pickle-suckers tell you that you are wasting your time.

3. YOU WILL BE MORE RESILIENT

In his book *The Last Lecture* Randy Pausch wrote that brick walls are not there to stop you, they are there to make you prove how much you want something. You do not prove how much you want something by complaining about it, you prove how much you want it by taking action. Bad things do happen to good people; making The Pickle Pledge a part of your philosophical DNA will help you plow through those brick walls instead of being stopped by them.

4. YOU WILL BE A BETTER PARENT

The biggest impact you will have on your children will not be what you say to them or what you give to them – it will be the example that you set for them. The more they hear you complain about how much you dislike your odious job, the more likely it is that they will grow up with their own negative attitudes about the meaning of work. You run the risk of raising Junior Dilberts who will end up dead-ended in dead-end jobs because they are competing with other people who are passionate about work – and who are committed to turning complaints into blessings and constructive suggestions rather than just whining about them. Teaching your kids to internalize The Pickle Pledge – especially through your example – will be one of the greatest gifts that you can give to them.

5. YOU WILL BE A BETTER FRIEND

Sometimes the best friends are those who, rather than commiserating with us about our complaints (remember, when you break the work commiserate down you get co-miserate: to be miserable together) help us to look up, buck up, and shape up. They will listen to your complaint, but instead of reinforcing your sense of victimhood they inspire you to grow up and deal with it.

6. YOU WILL BE A BETTER CAREGIVER

You cannot be a negative, bitter, cynical sarcastic pickle-sucker in the break room and then somehow magically flip a switch and become a genuinely caring and compassionate caregiver when you walk into a patient's (or in long-term care a resident's) room. And people very quickly tell the difference.

7. YOU WILL BE A BETTER MANAGER AND A BETTER LEADER

One definition holds that management is doing things right and leadership is doing the right thing. Complaining, and commiserating with those who complain, does not fit either definition.

8. YOU WILL BE MORE PRODUCTIVE

What can be a bigger waste of time than complaining? And not only does it waste the precious moments during which you are actually engaged in whining, it puts you into a more depressive state of mind that diminishes your productivity in the moments and hours to come.

9. You will be wealthier

When you make the commitment to turn complaints into constructive suggestions you begin to see opportunities where before you saw only barriers. This will make you more valuable, and thus more likely to be promoted, at work. You will gain a reputation as a problem-solver, and thus more likely to have others seeking you out for even better-paying jobs. And you will spend less and save more, partly because complaining is depressing and many of us deal with depression by indulging in shopping therapy.

10. You will be happier

By definition people do not complain about things that make them happy. The more you complain the more you are focusing your precious life's energy on things that make you unhappy. A big part of the magic of The Pickle Pledge is that just by saying the words you will inevitably change your mindset. Smile from the outside in for long enough and pretty soon you'll be smiling from the inside out.

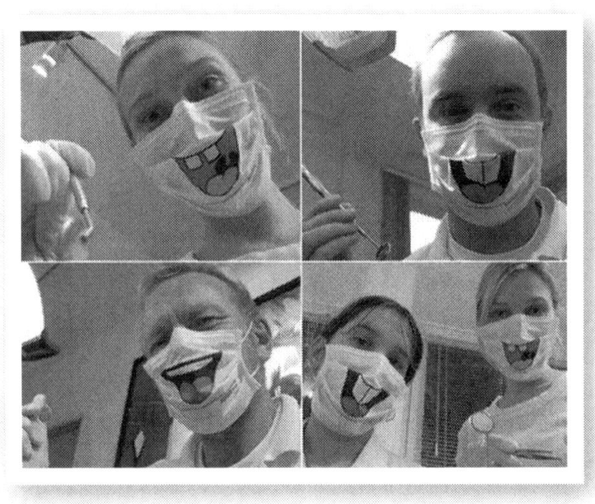

YOU CAN REWIRE YOUR BRAIN

One of the most exciting fields of neuroscience today is that of brain plasticity – the ability of the human mind to reconfigure its internal wiring in response to experience and thought. This has tremendous implications for making a daily commitment to reciting The Pickle Pledge (including the footnote). Do this often enough and for long enough and you will be hardwiring your brain for positive thinking. In other words, by changing the software of the words you use you can actually change the hardware of the brain that processes those words.

> *"[W]e are seeing evidence of the brain's ability to remake itself throughout adult life, not only in response to outside stimuli, but even in response to directed mental effort. We are seeing, in short, the brain's potential to correct its own flaws and enhance its own capabilities."*
>
> Jeffrey M. Schwartz, M.D. and Sharon Begley: *The Mind and the Brain: Neuroplasticity and the Power of Mental Force*

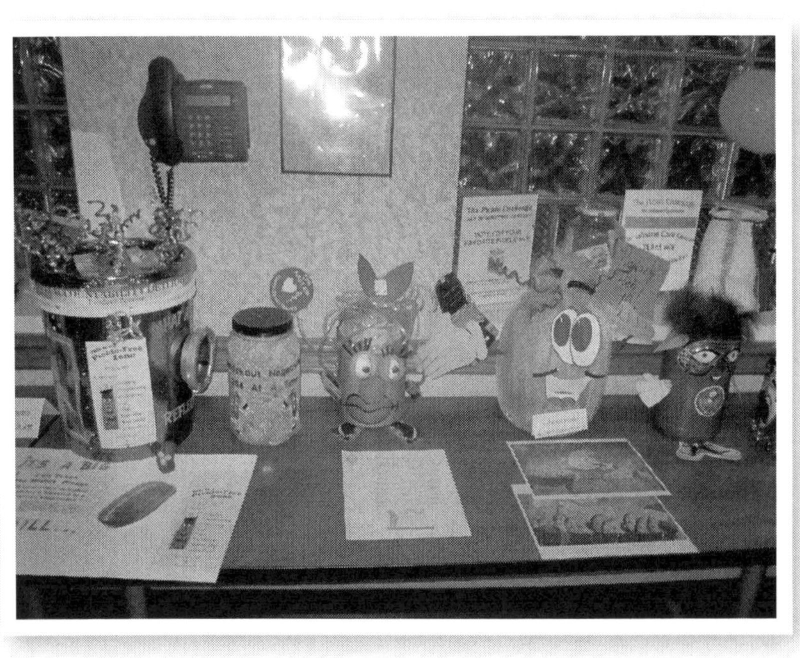

THE POWER OF CUES

There have been a number of books recently covering the art and science of habit change (e.g. *The Power of Habit* by Charles Duhigg, *Triggers* by Marshall Goldsmith, and *Nudge* by Richard Thaler and Cass Sunstein). One consistent theme across all of this research is the importance, and the power, of visual reminders. Keeping The Pickle Pledge, and Pickle-Free Zone signs and door hangers, where you will see them often will help you shift your attitude – and also serve notice on others that you will not allow them to waste your time and energy with their negative attitudes.

A business office employee reported that every day after lunch a coworker would stop by her cubicle and dump the complaint of the day in her lap, then leave. She said that it was terribly depressing, and that it took her about half an hour to get back to being productive. So she posted a sign declaring her workspace a Pickle-Free Zone; when her coworker would skulk in after lunch with the complaint de jure, she would simply nod toward the sign. The coworker, evidently having nothing positive to talk about, doesn't come in any more. And the business office employee is happier and more productive.

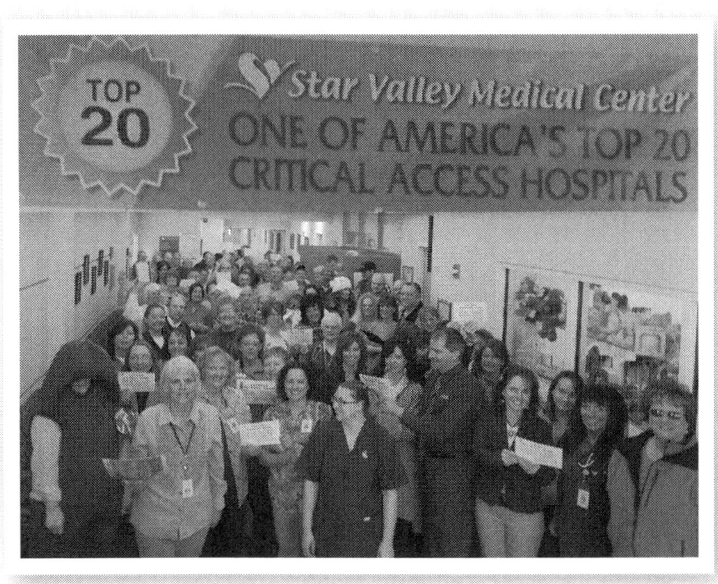
TOP 20
Star Valley Medical Center
ONE OF AMERICA'S TOP 20
CRITICAL ACCESS HOSPITALS

NATURE, NURTURE AND CHOICE

Psychologists have long debated, and parents often wonder, about the respective roles of nature and nurture. *Nature* is the genetic makeup you were born with. *Nurture* is the sum total of your lifetime experiences. They both have had a big impact on making you the person you are today.

But here's the deal: when it comes to your future, nature and nurture are both completely and totally meaningless! They can serve no other purpose than as an excuse to prevent you from taking action. Nature and nurture are the deadweight of the past. Choice is all that matters. You *can choose* what to do with the genes you were born with. You *can choose* how to interpret the experiences of your past.

If you were born with a disability you can choose to sit on the sidelines and feel sorry for yourself, or you can choose to find a way to lead a happy and productive life despite your limitations. If you were raised by an abusive parent you can choose to follow that role model and be an abusive parent yourself, or you can choose to become an advocate fighting on behalf of other abused children. You can choose to take the easy path and make excuses for why you are not more than you are, or you can choose to take the road less traveled and become the person you were meant to be. The choice is yours. The Pickle Pledge can help you choose wisely.

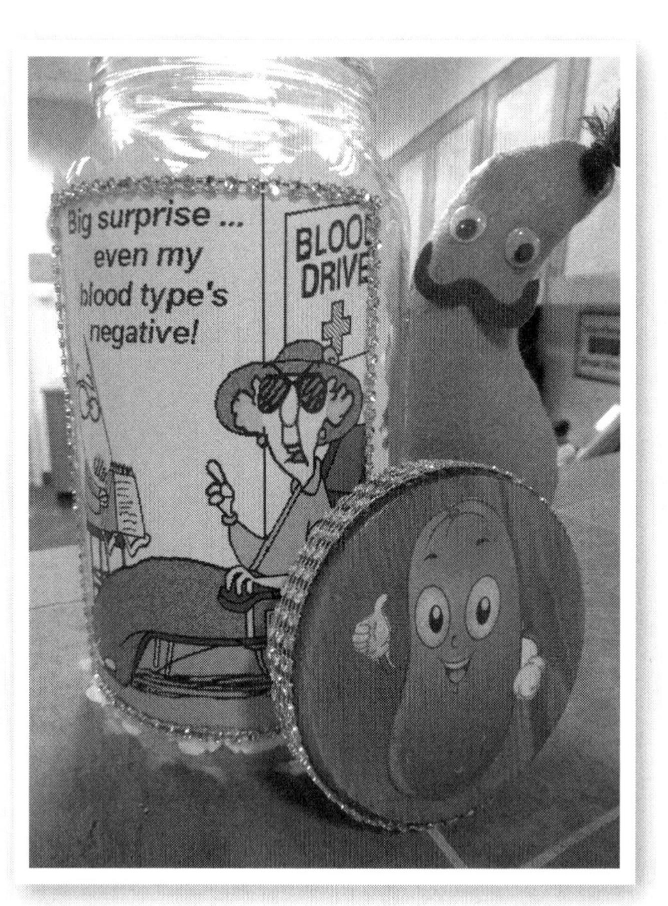
Big surprise ...
even my
blood type's
negative!
DRIVE

Complaining and the Paradox of Motivation

It's easy to be motivated when things are going great – it's also irrelevant because things are already going great. It's hardest to be motivated when things are falling apart, but that's also when motivation is most needed and when it has the greatest leverage. But if you wait until you need the motivation to start working on being a motivated person it might well be too late.

In a variation on the paradox of motivation, the times when renewal is most important are times of personal challenge and crisis. With a commitment to The Pickle Pledge the loss of a job, midlife crisis, financial or health challenges, or any other apparent adversity can be transformed into the opportunity for renewal and redirection. But the time to cultivate the necessary strength of character is *before* you are called upon to exercise it.

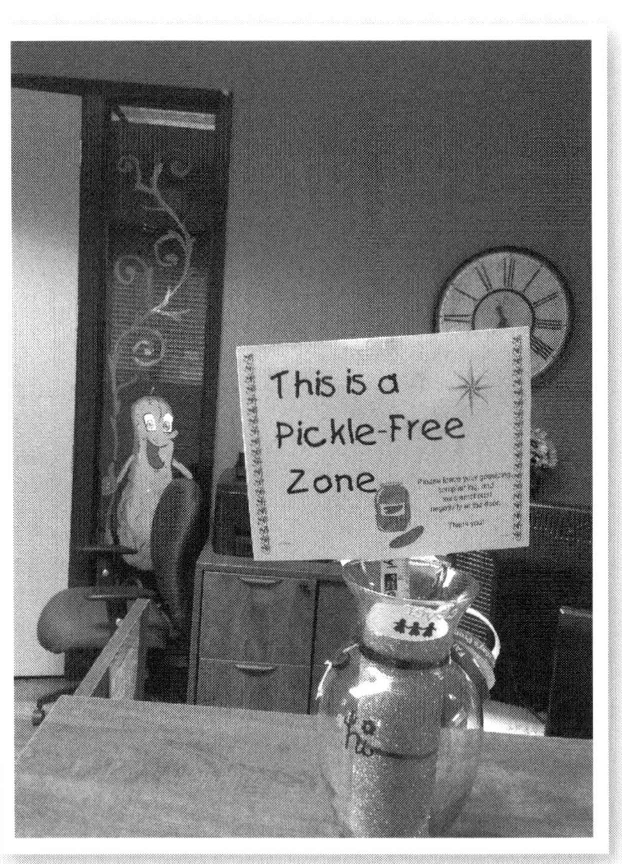
This is a
Pickle-Free
Zone

The Pickle Pledge Gives a New Language for Confronting Toxic Emotional Negativity

The Pickle Pledge gives people a lighthearted and soft touch language for confronting toxic emotional negativity. Instead of telling someone to "quit our bellyaching" you can simply invite them to deposit a quarter. They'll get the message.

We heard from one hospital nursing unit where everyone had given up on ever getting through to a nurse who was widely seen as a bullying emotional vampire, but who saw herself as a constructive critic. When she refused to participate in The Pickle Challenge for Charity, calling it "a stupid kindergarten game," her coworkers agreed to put a quarter in their pickle jar on her behalf every time this nurse engaged in toxic emotional negativity. Seeing how fast the pickle jar filled up with quarters deposited on her account by her nursing unit colleagues did more to influence her attitude than all of the words that had ever been spoken to her by managers and coworkers.

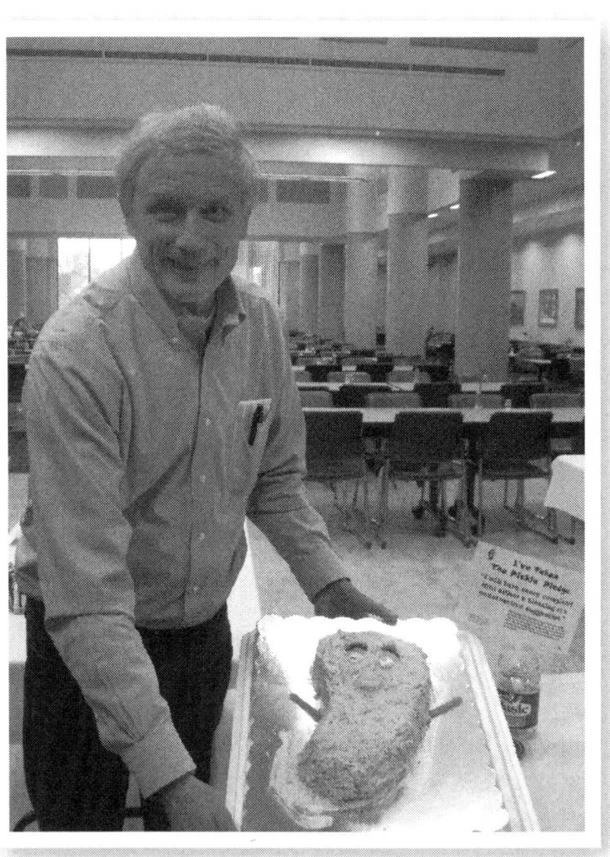

Imagine your workplace as a Pickle-Free Zone

Imagine a workplace where every time someone started to bitch, moan, whine or complain about something they would pull themselves up short, or were nudged by someone else to do so, and turned that complaint into a blessing and/or a constructive suggestion. How much more pleasant and less stressful would it be to work there? How much more productive would that workplace be? Think it's impossible? We're here to tell you that not only is it possible, it might be a whole lot easier than you think.

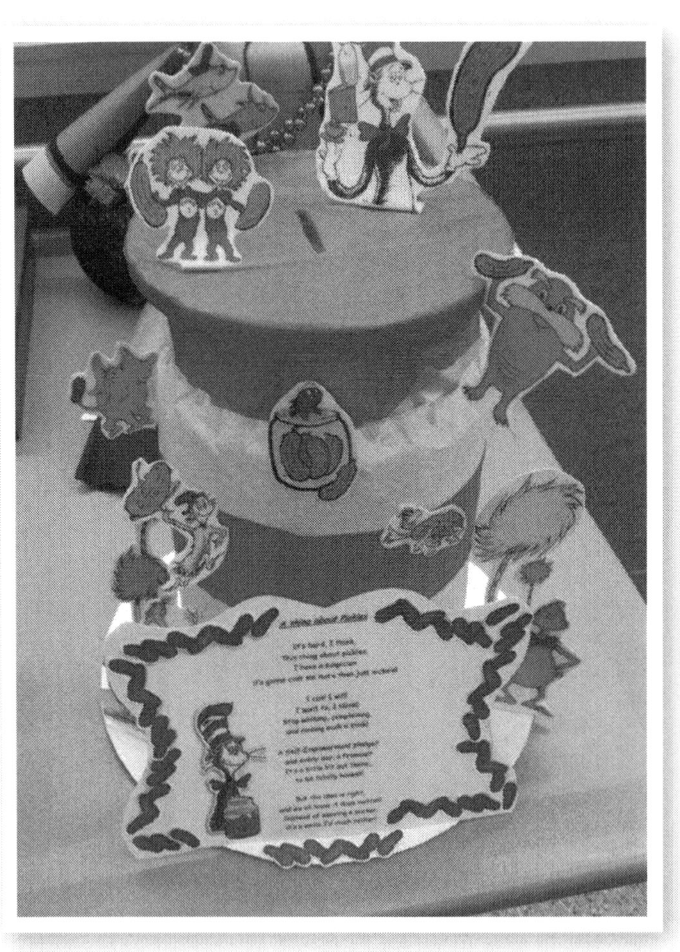

Imagine Yourself as a Pickle-Free Person

Question #1: If you personally were to take The Pickle Pledge to heart, would you be better off than where you are headed now – personally, professionally, financially, and spiritually?

Question #2: If everyone where you work made a good faith effort to take The Pickle Pledge to heart, would you do a better job of serving patients and of supporting each other?

If you are being honest with yourself, the answer to both questions will be Yes – absolutely!"

So the obvious next question is – Why don't we do it here in our organization? Why don't we make the collective commitment to The Pickle Pledge and promote a more positive and productive organization? All you need is a few brave souls to bring in a pickle jar, hang a sign on their door, and refuse to contribute to or participate in toxic emotional negativity. You need to stand solidly behind them when they are criticized or ridiculed by the pickle-suckers who don't want to see positive change. Join the movement yourself by taking The Pickle Pledge to heart, putting your quarters in the pickle jar, and hanging a pickle-free door hangar on your office door. And set a positive example by being a Spark Plug yourself.

A hospital nurse went home at the end of her shift one day and saw a handmade copy of The Pickle Pledge lying on her kitchen table, obviously the work of her seventh grade daughter. She recognized it immediately because they had taken The Pickle Challenge for Charity at her hospital, but she herself had not brought it home with her. It turned out that the daughter of another hospital employee had taken it to her house and shared it with her family. That daughter had taken it in and shared it with the teacher, who in turn gave it to the rest of the class as a project. And that is how the movement spreads.

Part 5
The Pickle Challenge for Charity

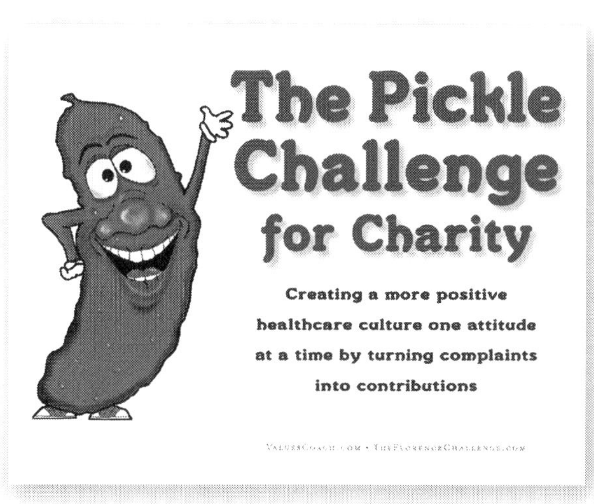

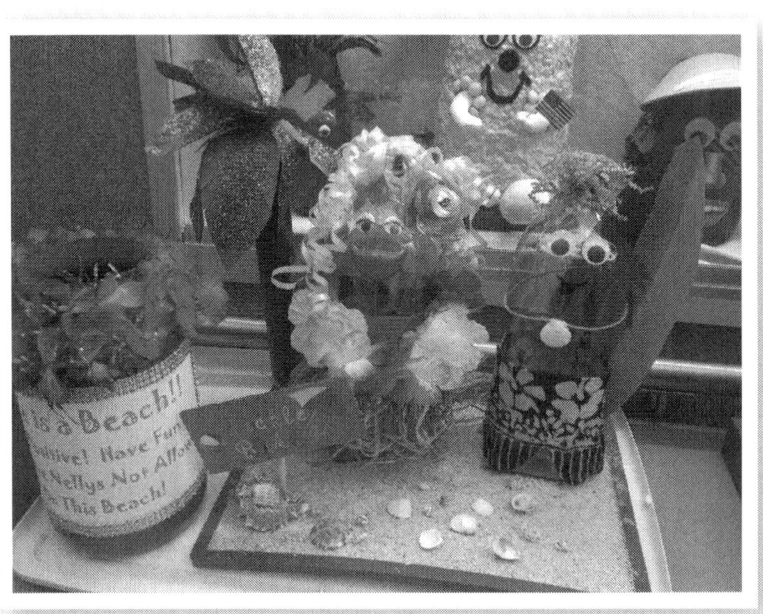
is a Beach!!
Have Fun
Nellys Not
This Beach!

CHANGING CULTURE ONE ATTITUDE AT A TIME

The Pickle Challenge for Charity is a fun and lighthearted way for people to catch themselves, and each other, complaining and to serve up a reminder that buried within that complaint there is a blessing and/or a constructive suggestion. Remember: Culture does not change unless and until people change, and people will not change unless given the tools and structure and inspired by values.

This really works!

The first 16 Values Coach clients that took The Pickle Challenge for Charity collectively raised more than $20,000 during their one-week challenge periods. Now think about that for a minute. In these 16 organizations in just a one-week period, more than 80,000 quarters were deposited in pickle jars. That means that more than 80,000 times during that one-week period – *in just those 16 organizations!* – people called themselves or their coworkers out for exhibiting negative attitudes and behaviors. With matching donations from Values Coach and others, more than $30,000 was raised for charities during that one week period – *in just those 16 organizations!*

Extrapolating those results to a full year, in just those 16 organizations, more than 4 million episodes of TEN would have been transformed into more positive behaviors such as spending time with patients, communicating with other departments, investing in personal education and development. Extrapolating those results to the entire healthcare system suggests that if every organization were to take The Pickle Challenge for a year, *more than one billion* episodes of TEN could be transformed into positive and productive activity. Extrapolating to our society overall suggests that five to ten billion times a year people engage in various forms of TEN. Imagine the impact upon our organizations, our families and communities, and our world if those billions of complaints were to be transformed into positive expressions of gratitude and commitments to take action – and contributions to worthy causes.

These behaviors diminish self-respect; foster unhealthy relationships; and impair performance, customer service, and productivity of organizations. They have no place in healthcare organizations.

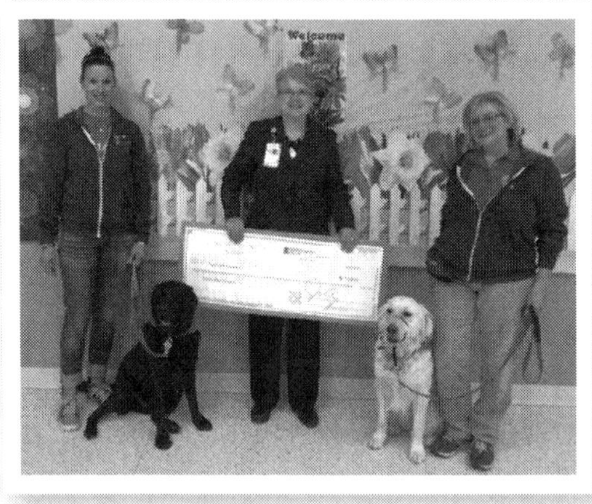

Commandant Jodi Tymeson of the Iowa Veterans Home with the Values Coach matching donation to their charity of choice – a nonprofit organization that trains service dogs

What you expect and what you tolerate

The emotional climate of the workplace will be determined by what you expect and what you tolerate, and over time what you tolerate will dominate what you say you expect.

If the words on the wall say that you expect integrity, but your culture tolerates two people talking about a coworker behind that person's back, then you have lowered the bar on what you mean by integrity.

If the words on the wall say that you expect great customer service, but your culture tolerates patients overhearing complaining on the part of employees, then you have lowered the bar on what you mean by excellence.

The Pickle Challenge for Charity raises intolerance for attitudes and behaviors that should not – that must not! – be tolerated in a healthcare organization.

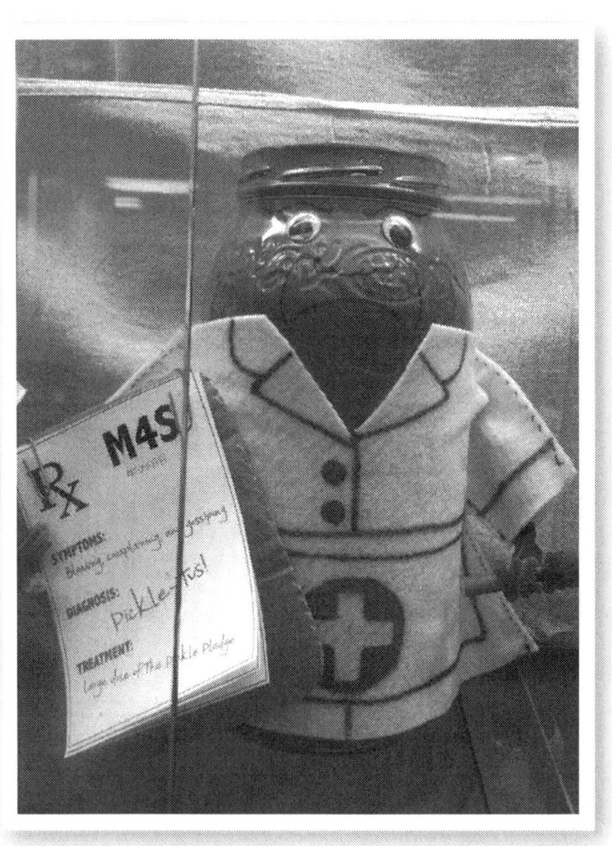
M4S
Rx
SYMPTOMS:
DIAGNOSIS:
TREATMENT:

Making Cultural Transformation Fun

The Pickle Challenge for Charity will unleash incredible creativity. The starting point is the pickle jar decorating contest. Every department and nursing unit is challenged to come up with a creative pickle jar for their 25-cent TEN deposits. Before official launch of The Challenge they are brought to a central location (typically the cafeteria) where people vote on their favorites. In many cases decorated pickle jars are maintained long after The Pickle Challenge for Charity has ended and the ritual of reminding people to mind their attitudes becomes part of that unit's cultural DNA.

"Ladies and Gentlemen, The Pickles"!
Pickle Free Zone
STOP THAT PICKLE!!!
STAY OUT OF THE BRINE ... Get rid of that whine.
SALTY
SOUR
SPICY
SCRAM!

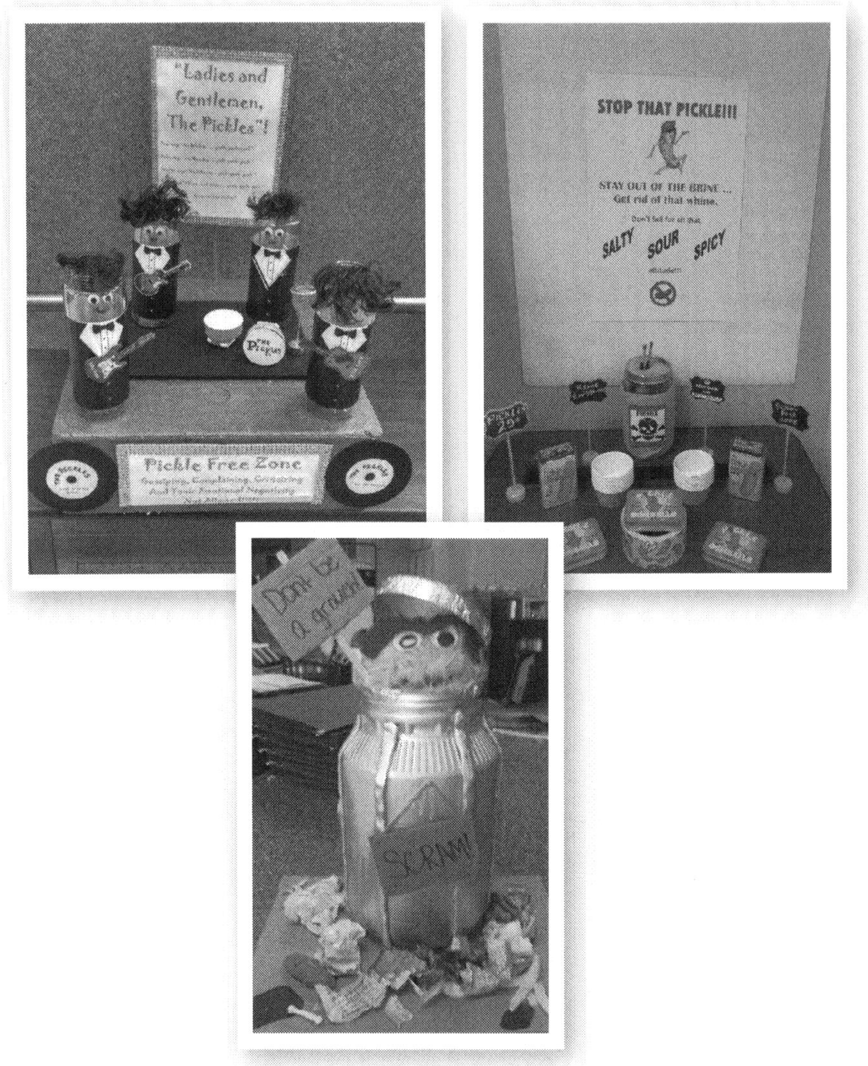

Examples of creatively decorated pickle jars from The Pickle Challenge for Charity

Note: You can see many more examples of some of the incredibly creative ways that people have promoted The Pickle Challenge for Charity, including a 3-minute video from Carilion Clinic, a large healthcare system in Roanoke, Virginia, at www.TheFlorenceChallenge.com/Pickle.

From Accountability to Ownership

There are two possible approaches to eliminating toxic emotional negativity and replacing it with behaviors that reflect a more positive attitude: accountability or ownership. Accountability is imposed; ownership is inspired. Accountability is the approach of holding people's feet to the fire; ownership is the approach of inspiring people to walk across hot coals on their own. To a large extent, the two approaches are mutually exclusive. The more heavily you bring down the hammer of accountability, the harder it will be for you to foster a true culture of ownership.

When Joe speaks for the classes that Bob teaches at the University of Texas Permian Basin School of Nursing in Odessa, he plays a word association game with the students. He throws out the word "accountability." Students shout back words like rules, consequences, punishment, looking over your shoulder, April 15th and, yes, holding your feet to the fire. We've never once heard words like pride, passion, commitment or engagement being associated with the word accountability. Nobody will ever go home and brag to their children about having been held accountable at work.

The Pickle Pledge and The Pickle Challenge for Charity must be embraced voluntarily – they cannot be imposed hierarchically. But when people are invited – not instructed – to participate, you will be astonished at the creativity, passion, and ultimately commitment is generated. More important, you will be astonished by the way some of the people you considered to be irremediably negative will, as a result of seeing the quarters pile up, become more aware of their own attitudes and of how they are perceived by others. When they do, they make remarkable (and in some cases miraculous) turnarounds.

> *"Accountability is supposed to improve productivity by tracking performance. Up to a point, like most well-intended management expectations, this one may have the desired effect. In the long run, however, there could hardly be a more inhibiting practice. When made a fetish, accountability stifles creativity. Far from making employees perform better long term, accountability encourages a culture of evasion, denial, and finger pointing."*
>
> Richard Farson and Ralph Keyes: *The Innovation Paradox: The Success of Failure, the Failure of Success*

For more on the downside of trying to create a culture where performance is motivated by accountability rather than a spirit of ownership see Joe's article "Building a Culture of Ownership in Health Care" in the American Hospital Association publication *H&HN Daily* at this link: http://www.hhnmag.com/articles/4074-an-ownership-culture

Son, you'll be proud of your old Dad...
Today they held me accountable.

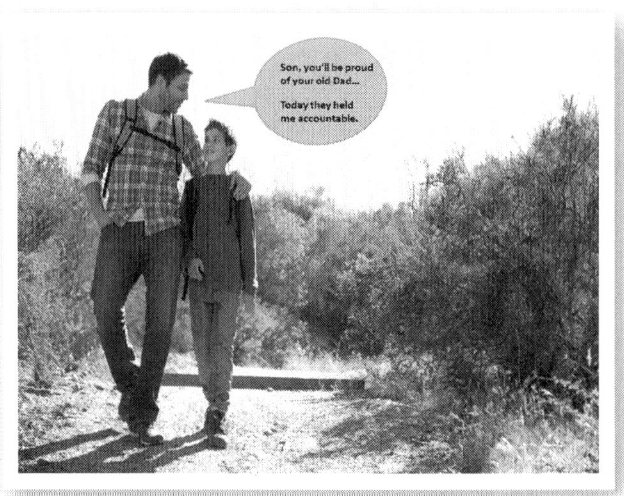

DAISY AWARDS ARE EARNED FOR ATTITUDE, NOT JUST SKILL

In *The Leadership Challenge*, James Kouzes and Barry Posner write, "Leaders give heart by visibly recognizing people's contributions to the common vision and letting others know how much they mean to the organization." One such way to recognize exemplary nurses is the DAISY Award® for Extraordinary Nurses (www.DaisyFoundation.org) At Midland Memorial Hospital, nurses who have been nominated by patients, family members or others and selected by a panel of peers are surprised with the recognition during a shift and celebrated by their colleagues. The person nominating them is often present to express their gratitude for the compassionate care they experienced by sharing his or her story and the impact felt as a result. These ceremonies are heartfelt and often emotional. MMH nurses proudly wear their DAISY pins on their badges, and the hospital prominently displays names and photographs of award-winners on the DAISY wall in a main thoroughfare of the hospital. They are recognized again during Nurses Week each year.

DAISY Nurses are recognized for their "above and beyond" compassion and skill. Their patients, and their patients' family members, feel their passion and their compassion every day. We have yet to see an emotional vampire or a pickle sucker be nominated for The DAISY Award. With DAISY Awards as with so much else in life, attitude really is everything.

There's an important side-note here. The antidote to what is pejoratively called "program of the month" syndrome is what Joe calls "initiative coherence" – making it clear how various "programs" build upon and reinforce one another. Midland Memorial Hospital is a better place to work and a better place to receive care *because* we have adopted multiple "programs" with those goals in mind.

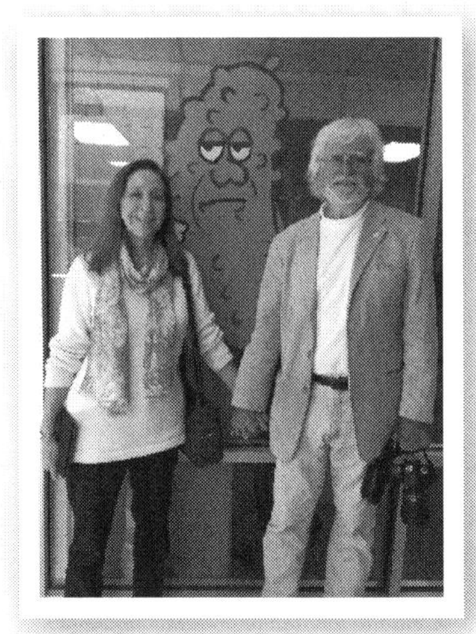

DAISY Foundation founders Mark and Bonnie Barnes with one of the many "pickle reminders" at Midland Memorial Hospital

Note: Values Coach Inc. is proud to be an honorary DAISY Foundation Partner and to have honored the DAISY Foundation with its INSPIRED Award for Values and Culture Excellence to recognize their contributions to helping hospitals and other healthcare organizations foster a more positive culture.

Coffee and Water

Fill two clear glass coffee cups half-full, one with water and the other with black coffee. Take a t-spoon of water and pour it into the coffee. The appearance of the coffee doesn't change at all, does it? Now take a t-spoon of coffee and pour it into the water. What happens? It is instantly discolored.

That's a great metaphor for what happens in the workplace. If you bring a positive person into a toxic negative environment, it won't be long before that person joins in with the complaining crowd, or simply withdraws or leaves the organization for a more positive experience elsewhere. On the other hand, if you inject a toxically negative individual into a previously positive workplace environment it won't be very long at all before that person begins to contaminate everyone he or she comes into contact with unless they have the courage to vote the negative newcomer off the island.

If the organization has a strong positive culture, that toxically negative individual will be rejected the way a body will reject a mismatched organ transplant. But if there's a weak culture, that previously clear glass will be permanently stained.

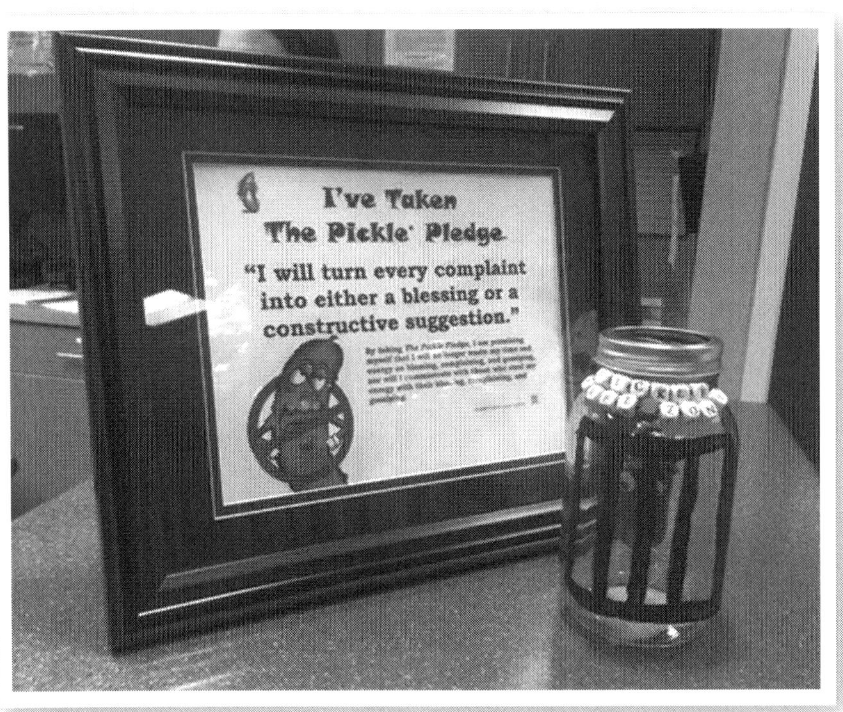
I've Taken
The Pickle Pledge
"I will turn every complaint into either a blessing or a constructive suggestion."

12 Key Success Factors

In analyzing the most effective examples we've seen of The Pickle Challenge for Charity in action, 12 strategies stand out.

1. Do an Objective Assessment and Take Off the Rose-Colored Glasses

Research by The University of Iowa Department of Health Management and Policy shows that the higher on the organization chart one's position is, the more likely they will be to view their culture through rose-colored glasses. An unpublished follow-up study shows a strong correlation between cultural clarity at every level of the organization and higher patient satisfaction and quality indicators (personal correspondence with lead investigator). No matter how positive you personally think you are, and no matter how great you think your culture is, if you really start paying attention to TEN you will be astonished, and appalled, at how prevalent it really is. When Values Coach works with healthcare clients, the first step is almost always to conduct a Culture Assessment Survey. This provides a unique window into how people actually perceive the elements of Invisible Architecture – core values, organizational culture, and workplace attitude – and allows comparison with a growing data base of other organizations. It also allows us to estimate the financial and personal cost of TEN in that organization.

2. Select a Great Charity and Solicit Matching Donations

Selecting a charity that many people will feel an emotional connection to helps give momentum to The Pickle Challenge. Engaging people in making the selection (something Joe does during kick-off leadership retreats when Values Coach is participating) helps foster a stronger sense of ownership. Values Coach often offers a partial matching donation and encourages the organization to recruit other matching donors, thus raising the stakes – and the motivation level – for successfully meeting The Challenge.

3. Set a Positive Leadership Example

The example set by the leadership team, including members of middle management, is crucial. It's not enough that managers be merely in favor or supportive of The Pickle Pledge and The Pickle Challenge for Charity – what's needed is the enthusiasm that goes with truly believing that something is important and that it will make a difference. At Midland Memorial Hospital, the CEO and every other member of the executive team wears their daily wristbands for the seven promises of The Self Empowerment Pledge and every morning one of them leads a large group in reciting both The Pickle Pledge and that day's promise from The Self Empowerment Pledge at the beginning of the Daily Leadership Huddle at the front entrance in the main lobby. For the letter C his book *Leadership A to Z: A Guide for the Appropriately Ambitious* James O'Toole chose the word "cheerleading" and asks why so many leaders forget this essential element of what it means to be a leader. Having managers as cheerleaders can make or break The Pickle Challenge for Charity.

4. Make it fun

Effective culture change must have more the feel of a social movement than that of a management program. The best way to gain widespread engagement and ownership is to make it fun, and even a bit silly. One of the ten core values at Zappos – which has turned teaching others about its culture into a profit center – is "Create fun and a little weirdness." That's what The Pickle Challenge for Charity does – gives people permission to have fun and be creative while challenging themselves and coworkers to be more positive, beginning with pre-Challenge activities such as pickle jar decorating and cake making contests.

5. Make it easy to participate

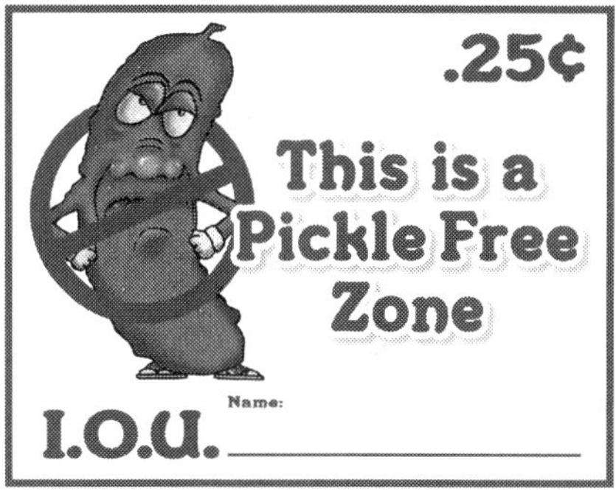

Recognizing that not everyone carries coins with them at work, consider providing an IOU form (one can be downloaded from www.TheFlorenceChallenge.com/Pickle), having a candy bowl with a supply of quarters as a loan fund, or other ways to allow people to participate if they don't happen to have a quarter handy when they catch themselves, or are caught by others, whining and complaining.

6. Have lots of visible reminders

At Midland Memorial Hospital you see pickles everywhere. There are decorated pickle jars in most departments, and for special events the food service department will make Pickle Pledge cakes and cupcakes. After a storm knocked down a big tree, one MMH employee turned a 2,000-pound tree stump into a chainsaw carving that now stands in a main thoroughfare of the hospital for employees, medical staff, and visitors to see, reminding people to leave their bad attitudes in the parking lot.

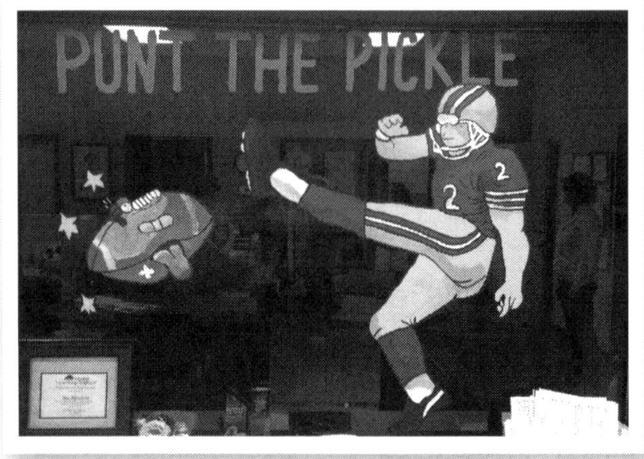

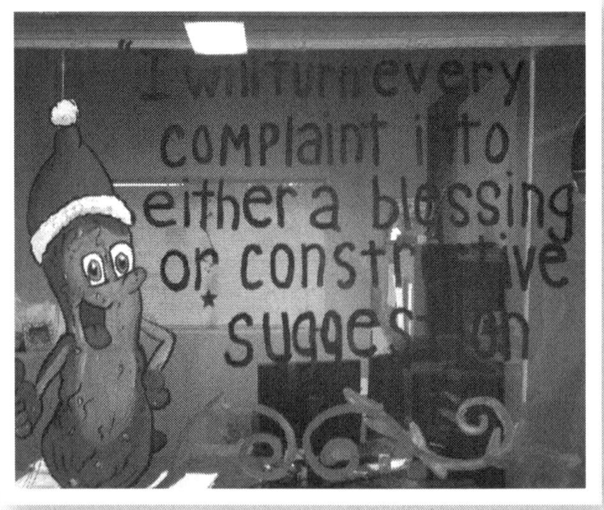

Keeping it visible at Kalispell Regional Healthcare in Kalispell, Montana

7. Unleash people's creativity

One of the most effective ways of launching The Pickle Challenge is by having an organization-wide pickle jar decorating contest.

You will be astonished at the creative thought and design that goes into those pickle jars! We have also seen pickle cake baking contests, we've seen singing pickles and dancing pickles, pickle statues and pickle piñatas. The CNO of one of the Indiana University Health System hospitals sent Joe a pickle poem that had been written by a patient. The Pickle Challenge will uncover amazing creative talent, sometimes in the most unexpected places.

8. CREATE SOCIAL EVENTS

As an essential food group, pickles lend themselves to all sorts of fun activities including creative cooking contests, pickle eating challenges, trading dill for sweet pickles, celebrating a week (or a month) of being pickle-free, and decorating the cafeteria with pickle themes.

Don't Be A Pickle!
The Pickle Pledge
"I will turn every complaint into either a blessing or a constructive suggestion."

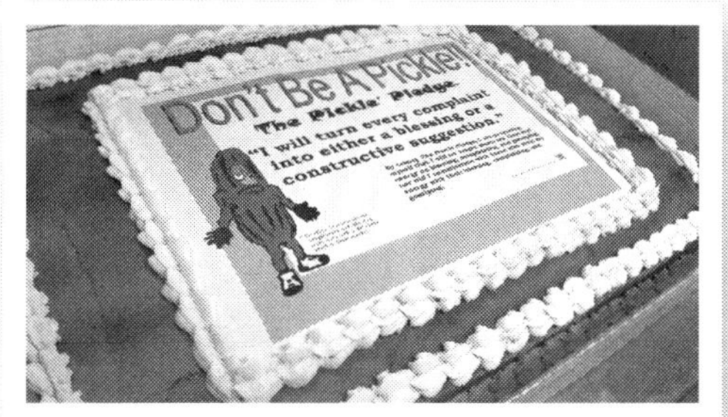

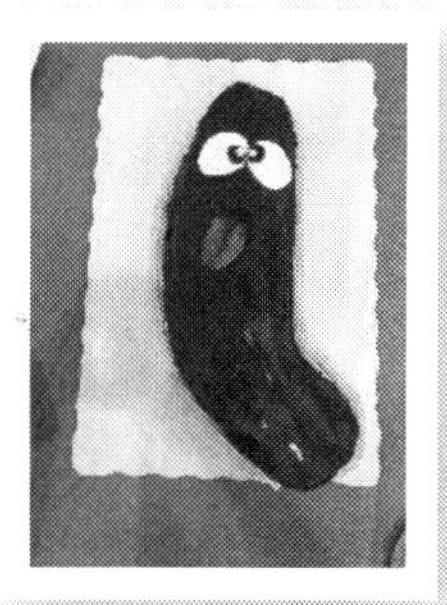

Examples of pickle cake-making contest entries

9. ENGAGE PATIENTS AND VISITORS

When patients go to the Patient Accounting department at Grinnell Regional Medical Center, they might have a complaint about their bill, but Penelope Pickle is there to remind them that rather than just complain about it, they should first be thankful for the excellent care they have received and then work on constructive solutions for dealing with the problem.

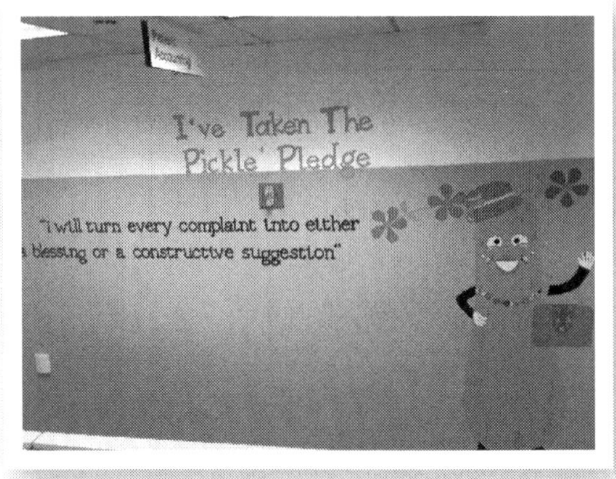

Penelope Pickle at Grinnell Regional Medical Center in Grinnell, Iowa

10. ENGAGE YOUR VOLUNTEERS

Volunteers love The Pickle Pledge – and can play an important role in fund-raising efforts in The Pickle Challenge for Charity. Because many volunteers have roles that are very public and visible, and are often out and about the facility, they are in a uniquely positive position to help promote the effort.

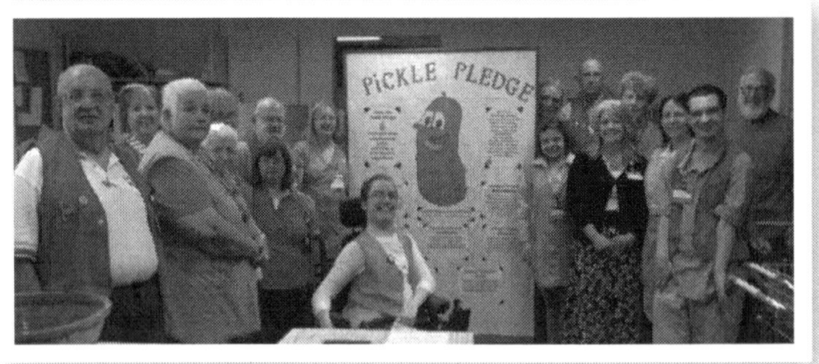

Volunteers at Guthrie Clinic in Sayre, Pennsylvania

11. Nurture and encourage your champions

It takes courage for someone to step up and be a "spark plug" for positive culture change – especially if that person has not historically been perceived as being a positive cheerleader. One of the most important duties of leadership – to encourage, honor, and protect those people who are trying to help foster a better organization by working at becoming better people.

12. Maintain momentum

It is absolutely predictable that any culture initiative, after an initial burst of enthusiasm, will run into resistance. This is where leadership is most severely tested. There will be a temptation to back off, to move on to other priorities. But backsliding will only contribute to the assertion of the cynics that this was just one more "program of the month." It is essential that the leadership team stay focused on defining and reinforcing the desired attitudes and behaviors until they have become part of the organization's cultural DNA – and then reach out to the broader community to foster a more positive overall culture. This might well be the most important lesson of the MMH experience: using the steps outlined above gives people clearly defined actions to help them stay focused on fostering a more positive culture of ownership.

** This section adapted from the article "The Pickle Challenge for a More Positive and Productive Culture" by Joe Tye in* Arkansas Hospitals, *Winter 2015*

One day a man came into his department, dropped a dollar bill into their decorated pickle jar, and said "I know it's going to be a shitty day, here's a buck – I'm paying in advance." He ended up having a great day because instead of the previous passive-aggressive response – Old Harry is having a bad day, give him a wide berth – they laughed and talked about it. He did not get a refund, but he did have a great day.

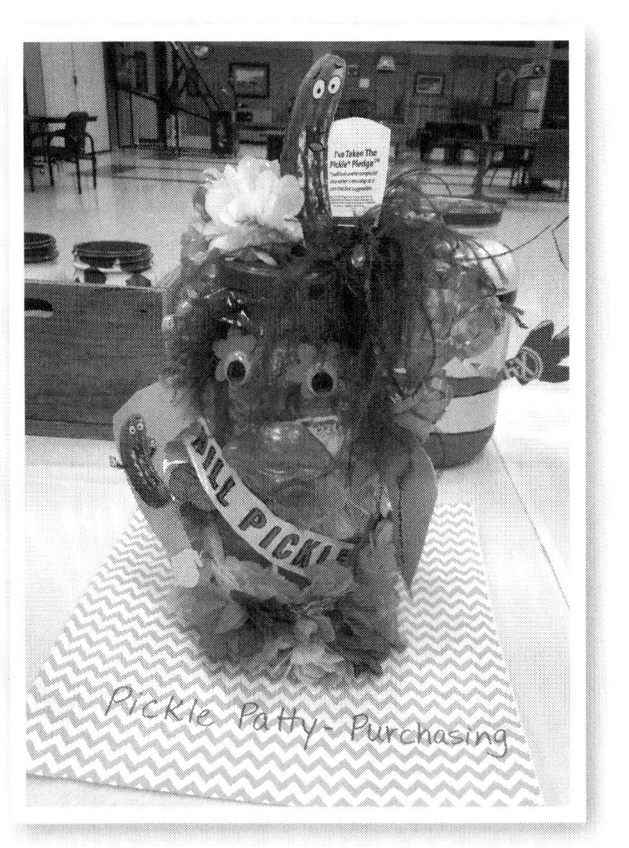
I've Taken The
Pickle® Pledge™
PICKLE
Pickle Patty- Purchasing

ANTICIPATE AND PREPARE FOR RESISTANCE

You will almost certainly get resistance to The Pickle Challenge for Charity, and it will be most vociferous from people who are the biggest part of the problem. In many cases, it will also be the people who could most benefit personally from having a more positive attitude – not to mention their families at home who receive the tail-end of toxic emotional negativity when Mom or Dad comes home at the end of a work day. Stick with it. While we can't promise this will happen, in many cases some of the people who are initially the most negative will end up being your most positive Spark Plugs as they experience the personal, professional and family benefits of taking The Pickle Pledge to heart.

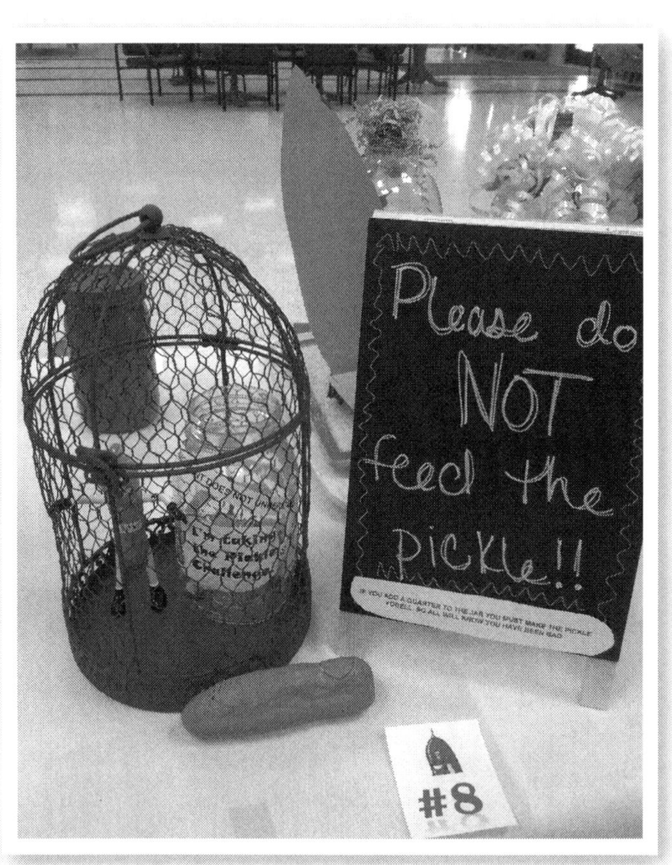
Please do NOT feed the PICKLE!!
#8

START A MOVEMENT!

Have you seen the TED Talk "How to Start a Movement" by Derek Sivers? As of this writing more than five and one-half million people have. In it, Sivers narrates an amateur video taken at an outdoor music festival. It starts with a man wearing no shirt or shoes dancing exuberantly in the grass – and being ignored by everyone around him. But then another man joins in, and almost immediately waves for three of his friends to come along. Over the next two minutes we see a movement blossom as hundreds of people jump up, join in and dance in the sunshine.

Sivers points out that, though after the fact he is considered the leader who started this movement, until he had attracted his first follower he was just "a lone nut" – a shirtless dancing guy at a concert. It was the first follower who transformed this lone nut into a leader.

There is a great lesson there for The Pickle Challenge for Charity. The first people to embrace it might be – okay, let's be honest, in all likelihood will be – considered lone nuts at first. That's why it's so important to have as many first followers join them as quickly as possible, helping the movement to reach a critical mass where it becomes unstoppable – like hundreds of people dancing in the sunshine at an outdoor music concert.

It takes courage to be the "lone nut" who starts a movement. It takes courage to be the first followers who help that movement gain traction. It takes courage for a manager to protect their lone nuts and first followers from the emotional vampires and pickle-suckers who want to kill the movement before it becomes part of the cultural DNA.

Fear is a reaction, courage is a decision. And perseverance is making that decision every day, day after day. Sustained courage will determine whether The Pickle Challenge for Charity helps you build a more positive and productive culture of ownership or becomes just one more "program of the month" that came and went without leaving a lasting legacy.

> *"It is not the law of large numbers or critical mass that creates change, but the presence of a small disturbance that gets into the system and is then amplified through the networks. Once inside the network, this small disturbance circulates and feeds back on itself. As different parts of the system get hold of it, interpret it, and change it, the disturbance grows. Finally, it becomes so amplified that it cannot be ignored."*
>
> Margaret Wheately: *Leadership and the New Science: Discovering Order in a Chaotic World*

The Triple Win

Fostering a stronger culture of ownership is a triple win. Patients win by being cared for in a more positive emotional environment, with more attention from caregivers and fewer errors in care delivery. Staff win by not being emotionally polluted with TEN during their work shift, and being able to go home to their families without taking workplace TEN home with them. And the organization wins with measurably enhanced productivity, patient satisfaction, and employee engagement.

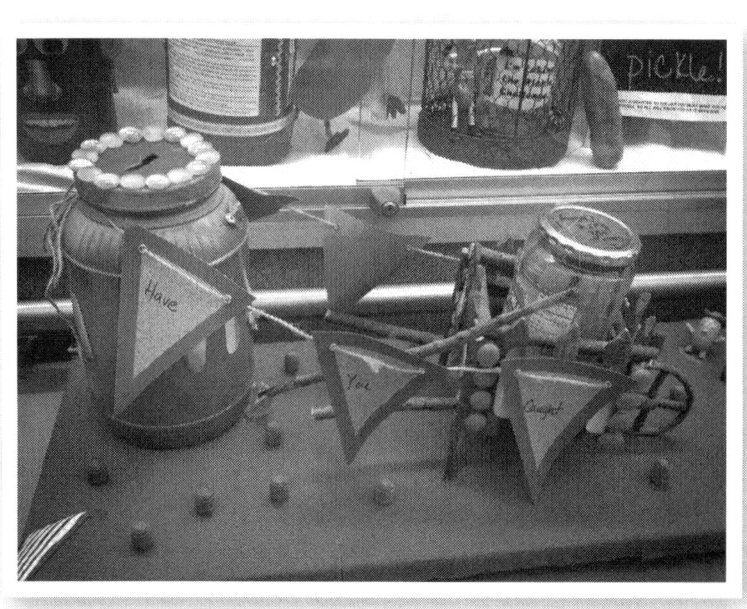
pickle!
Have
You
Caught

IF WE COULD WAVE A MAGIC WAND...

Are you old enough to remember when people smoked everywhere? When you couldn't see across the hospital cafeteria because of the smoky haze? When nurses smoked at the nurses' station and would light a patient's cigarette when they were sitting up in bed? When the "no smoking" light went out on an airplane you had to helplessly sit by and watch as people around you poisoned you (and your children) with their toxic cigarette smoke? If you are under the age of 30 you no doubt are having a hard time believing that this ever occurred but it's true.

When in 1986 Dr. C. Everett Koop declared the goal of a smoke-free society many people wondered what he'd been smoking! It was, after all, a long-enculturated practice that most people had grown to accept even if they didn't like or approve of it. The fact that nicotine is an addictive drug that is hard as heroin for many smokers to quit lent to the argument that we'd never achieve a tobacco-free world. And, of course, a whole industry of white collar drug pushers spent billions of dollars to promote cigarette smoking and what they called "smokers' rights."

Today, Dr. Koop's dream has been almost totally realized. Chances are good that you can go the rest of your life without having to inhale toxic cigarette smoke from someone else's cigarette. Anyone lighting a cigarette on an airplane would immediately be shown the door by fellow passengers. Almost all healthcare organizations prohibit smoking everywhere on their campuses. The chances that we will ever go back to allowing people to smoke cigarettes in public places are precisely ZERO because we all appreciate how much nicer life is when we (and our children) are not being poisoned by toxic smoke.

It will be the same thing with toxic emotional negativity in your workplace. As you work on building a more emotionally positive workplace culture – one where people do not tolerate chronic complaining, petty backbiting, gossip and rumor-mongering – you will never go back. If we could wave a magic wand over your facility – or over your entire community – and for one month it would be a Pickle-Free Zone (PFZ) the change would be permanent.

IMAGINE A SUPPORT GROUP WORKPLACE

One of the eight essential characteristics described in Joe's book *The Florence Prescription: From Accountability to Ownership* is a spirit of fellowship. If you have ever participated in a support group of any kind you have no doubt seen this spirit in action. People come together carrying heavy burdens – they have cancer, they are addicted to alcohol or drugs, they have suffered heartbreaking losses – but for several hours they can come together and help one another cope. Cope – not complain. When the meeting is over, they still have cancer, they are still addicts, what they have lost has not come back to them. But they have a little more hope, a little more courage, and a few more friends than they did before the meeting started.

Why can't the workplace be like that? Why can't, at the end of the day, people go home physically tired because they have been working hard, mentally drained because they have been thinking hard, but emotionally and spiritually uplifted because of the fellowship they've experienced throughout the day. The answer, of course, is that they can. All it takes is the courage to stop complaining and to start being thankful for the blessings in our lives and devoting ourselves to finding constructive suggestions for the problems we face. In short, to take to heart The Pickle Pledge.

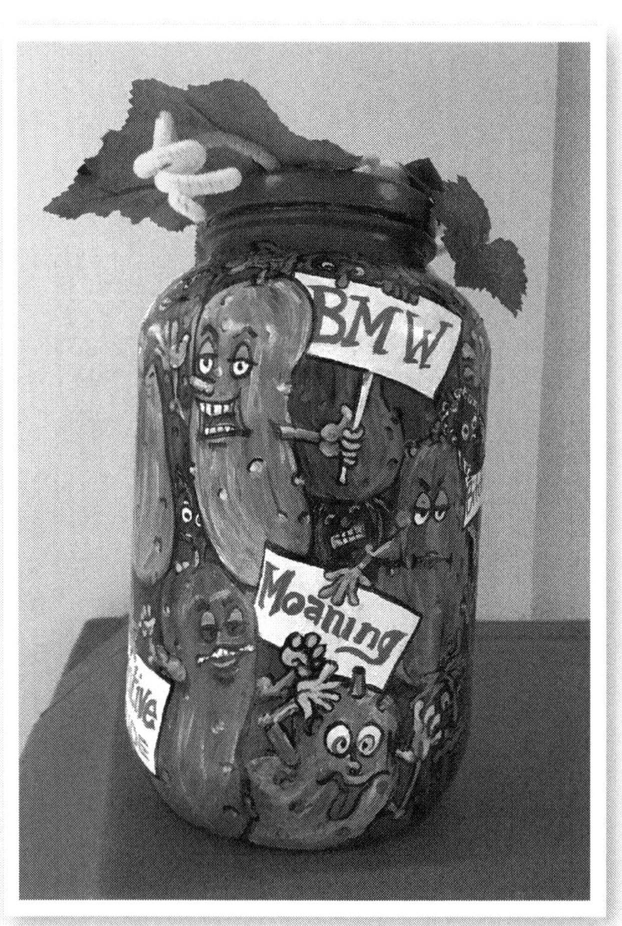
BMW
Moaning

And one last thing:

THE THOUGHT NOT TAKEN

By Joe Tye (with apologies to Robert Frost)

TWO thoughts converged between my ears,
I could not hang on to both;
One made me smile, the other brought tears
And dragged me backwards through the years
To sad memories of my youth.

That other thought cried and whined and moaned,
That life was so unfair,
At every inconvenience groaned,
With every complaint a mindful life postponed
The glass half filled with air.

The other smiled in gratitude
For the glass half filled with water,
And faced the emptiness with fortitude
Having made the choice of attitude
Knowing happiness is that choice's daughter.

I tell you this for lesson learned
Deadly as the Reaper's Scythe;
The complainer's road is dark and churned,
Littered with petty grievances unearned;
I chose to take the brighter path – and that has changed my life.

Part 6
About Values Coach

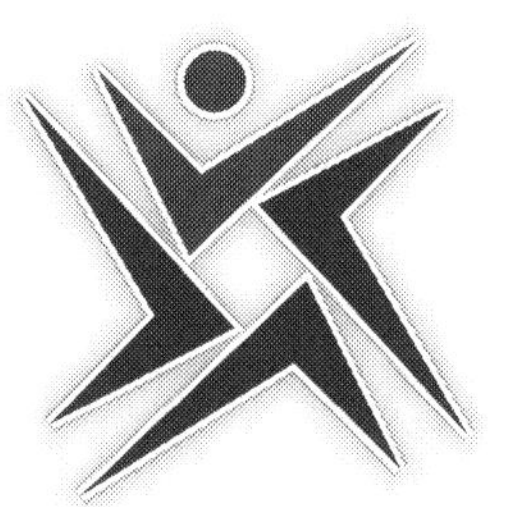

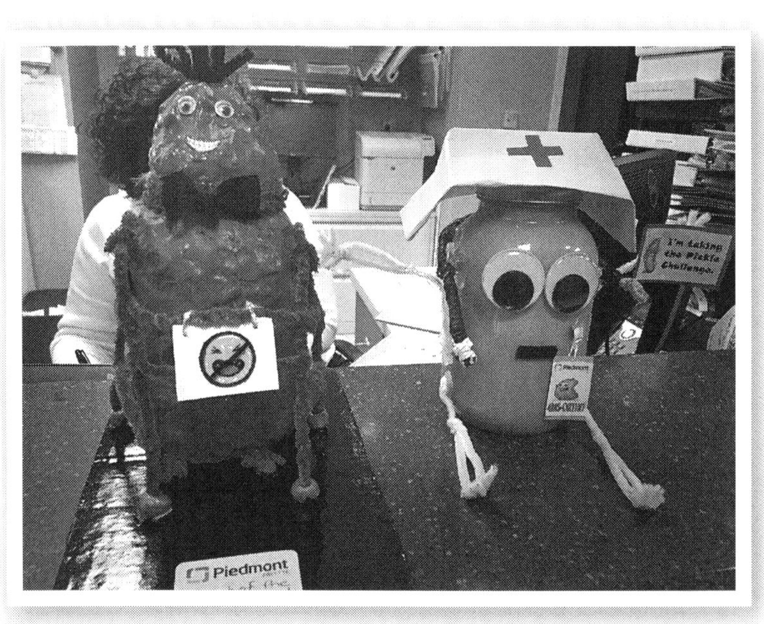
I'm taking the Pickle Challenge.
Piedmont

SUPPORT FROM VALUES COACH

You have blanket permission from Values Coach to use the ideas and program described in this book at no cost. This includes The Pickle Pledge and Pickle-Free Zone mini-poster and resources for The Pickle Challenge for Charity. You also have blanket permission to launch The Pickle Challenge for Charity in your organization at no cost – though we do request that you let us know you've started and what your final totals are by sending an email to Michelle@ValuesCoach.com.

In order to achieve optimal impact, however, we recommend that you have Values Coach support your effort with The Pickle Challenge Toolbox, which includes:

» Initial conference call and email support

» Values Coach will conduct before and after Culture Assessment Surveys and provide a consultation report with observations, comparisons with their growing data base of results, and recommendations for follow-up.

» A short introductory video by Joe Tye plus a customizable Power Point presentation that your manager can use to launch The Challenge in their area of responsibility; this will include slides with results of your organization's initial

Culture Assessment Survey including, where appropriate, Joe's commentary.

- Template for employee announcement, media release, and other helpful documents.
- Downloadable and shareable eBook edition of this book – Pickle Pledge.
- Downloadable and shareable 45-minute webinar on using The Pickle Pledge and The Pickle Challenge for Charity to promote a more positive and productive culture of ownership.
- Ongoing email consulting support.

To learn more about this toolbox, send an email to Michelle@ValuesCoach.com.

At the Values Coach store, Pickle-Free Zone door hangers are available for $1 apiece.

Helping Organizations Build a Culture of Ownership

Bring Joe Tye to Your Organization for a keynote, leadership retreat, all-employee assembly, or special event. Joe will inform and inspire your people.

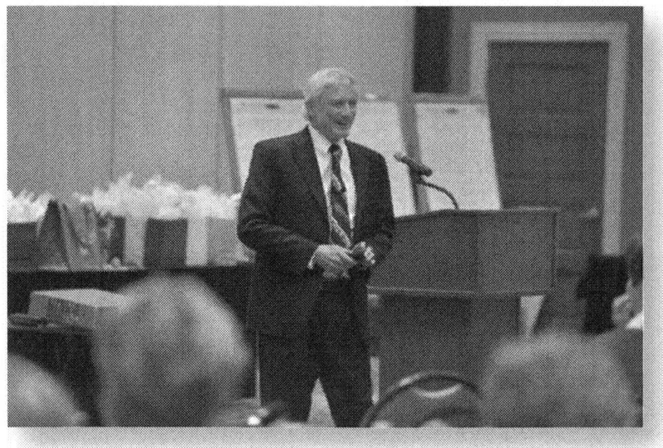

Visit www.ValuesCoach.com/speaking-topics for additional information

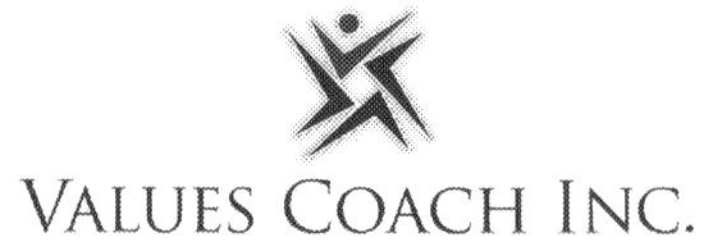

Values Coach Inc.

www.ValuesCoach.com

Michelle@ValuesCoach.com

319-624-3889

The INSPIRED Award for Honoring Values and Culture Excellence in Healthcare

The Values Coach INSPIRED Award for Values and Culture Excellence is awarded to healthcare organizations that have defined and implemented a process for blueprinting their Invisible Architecture™ of core values, organizational culture, and workplace attitude and promoted a more positive and productive culture of ownership.

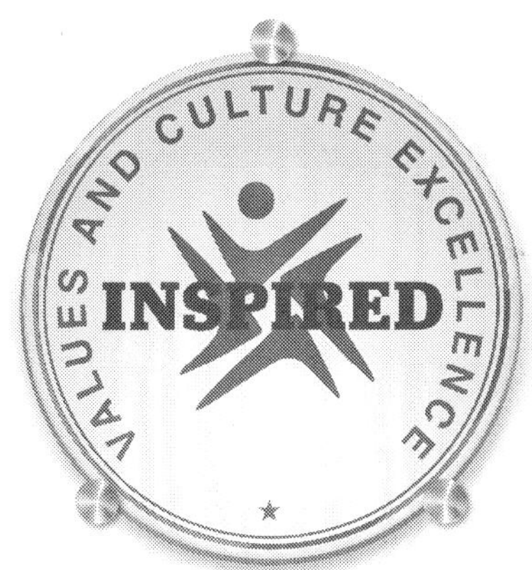

Download The INSPIRED Award for Values and Culture Excellent Flyer at www.ValuesCoach.com/build-a-culture-of-ownership

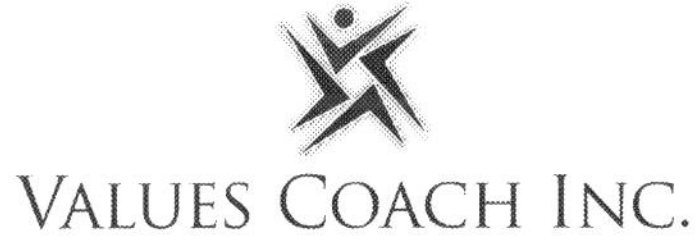

VALUES COACH INC.

www.ValuesCoach.com
Michelle@ValuesCoach.com
319-624-3889

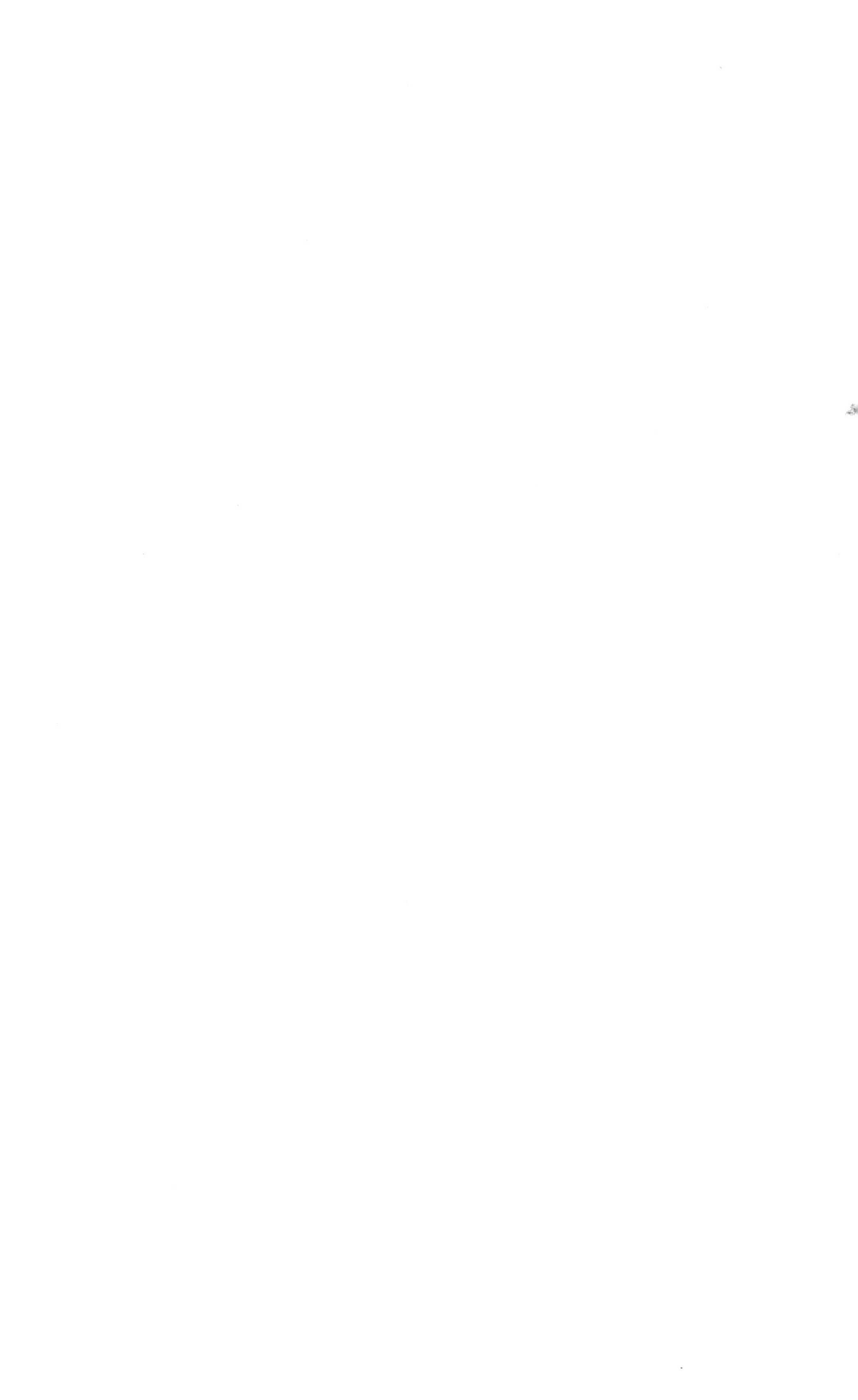

Made in the USA
Columbia, SC
01 May 2018